CLINICAL HANDBOOK
of Behavior Therapy

Adult Medical Disorders

Gerald Tarlow, Ph.D.

BROOKLINE
BOOKS

Library of Congress Cataloging-in-Publication Data

Tarlow Gerald.
Clinical handbook of behavior therapy.

Includes bibliographies and indexes.
Contents: v. 1. Adult medical disorders.
1. Behavior therapy—Handbooks, manuals, etc.
2. Cognitive therapy—Handbooks, manuals, etc.
I. Title. [DNDM: 1. Behavior Therapy. 2. Behavioral Medicine—methods. 3. Mental Disorders—therapy. WM 425 TI88c]
RC489.B4T37 1988 616.89'142 87-14634
ISBN 0-914797-89-5 (v. 1)

Published by
Brookline Books, Inc.
29 Ware Street
Cambridge, MA 02138

Table of Contents

Introduction

The major purpose of this book is to help the mental health clinician assess and treat a variety of problems by behavioral and cognitive-behavioral methods. The problems contained in this first volume are ones that may initially come to the attention of a physician, or may require a thorough physical evaluation, prior to treatment by a mental health clinician.

Each chapter in the book follows the same format. The section on assessment strategies suggests different strategies that have been employed, as discussed in the literature. Rating scales and some structured interviews are included in addition to behavioral observations. It is not the purpose of this section to teach differential diagnosis or review the diagnostic criteria of the disorders. The assessment techniques are generally ones that can best be used to assess the severity of a disorder or monitor treatment progress after a diagnosis has been confirmed.

The section on treatment strategies covers the successful behavioral treatments that have been reported in the literature. If a very simple, cost-effective treatment has been found to be effective, it will generally be reported first. Next, the techniques that have received the strongest support in the literature will be discussed. There is an emphasis on techniques that can be applied by the typical clinician. Techniques that require extensive apparatus are not emphasized. Additionally, biofeedback techniques are only briefly covered since many clinicians do not have access to the biofeedback equipment. There are excellent guidebooks available for the clinician interested in biofeedback, such as *Biofeedback: A Practitioner's Guide* (Schwartz, 1987). Techniques found to be unsuccessful are only briefly mentioned. This section does not evaluate the research that has been reported but suggests various treatment options that have been found to be successful, if even for two clinical case studies. Many chapters include detailed descriptions on how the techniques were applied in the research articles. It is also not the purpose of this book to teach basic behavior therapy techniques. There are many fine behavior therapy texts available, such as *Behavior Therapy Techniques and Empirical Findings* (Rimm & Masters, 1987).

The section at the end of each chapter, "For More Information," provides descriptions of key articles, book chapters, or entire books that would be useful if more in-depth knowledge is desired. Whenever possible the author's or publisher's address is included. The addresses were obtained from the article itself if it was published during the past two years. For older publications, the author's address was taken from the membership directory of the American Psychological Association, the membership directory of the Association for Advancement of Behavior Therapy, or the original article.

Each chapter has its own reference section and a cross reference to any other related chapters in this volume.

If the only reported research on a problem was unsuccessful, the problem was not included in the book. Also, some problems have been successfully treated in either one case study or in a series of case studies described in one article. These problem areas have been briefly summarized in Appendix A.

The effective use of the techniques in this book generally require more than just following the outlined procedures. It is important, of course, to develop a good relationship with the patient. Additionally, it is important to emphasize that the uniqueness of each patient, and the patient's environment, must be considered before applying the techniques in this book.

References

Rimm, D., & Masters, J. (1987). *Behavior therapy techniques and empirical findings*. New York: Academic Press.

Schwartz, M. (1987). *Biofeedback: A practitioner's guide*. New York: Guilford.

1 Anorexia Nervosa

Assessment Strategies

Any patient with symptoms of anorexia should have a complete physical exam prior to treatment. The physical exam will help to determine whether the patient requires inpatient hospitalization. For patients who can be treated on an outpatient basis, certain medical tests, for example, the measurement of electrolyte levels, should be done on a regular basis.

The initial behavioral assessment should last for one week. During this week the patient should be weighed daily, preferably first thing in the morning, under standardized conditions. Caloric intake and any episodes of bulimia also need to be monitored. In addition, during the baseline assessment week, obtain a list of potential reinforcers. The patient can complete the reinforcement survey schedule (Cautela & Kastenbaum, 1967) and keep track of all his or her activities during the week. Any high frequency behavior may be a potential reinforcer.

The Eating Attitudes Test (Garner & Garfinkel, 1979) can be given to the patient to obtain a measure of the symptoms in anorexia nervosa (Table 1-1).

Items marked with an "X" are scored 3 points and the adjacent responses are scored 2 points and 1 point, respectively. The mean score for a group of anorexia nervosa patients was 58.9 and for non-anoxerics was 15.6 (Garner and Garfinkel, 1979; 278).

It may also be necessary to observe the patient's eating behavior to assess any unusual eating habits (e.g., chopping food into very small pieces or food phobias). The Anorexic Behavioral Scale (Table 1-2) can help to identify behaviors that need to be further assessed and/or monitored.

When using the Anorexic Behavioral Scale, the examiner must judge whether the patient exhibits a particular behavior and mark Yes, No, or ?. A score of 2 is assigned when the behavior has definitely been observed, a score of 0 if it has definitely *not* been observed, and a score of 1 when there is some doubt in the rater's mind (Slade, 1973).

Good prognostic signs include no prior outpatient treatment, few anorexic behaviors, a good premorbid education, and vocational adjustment. Poor prognostic indicators include an excessive duration of the disorder, an older age at onset, severe weight loss, and bulimic behaviors. Many anorexic patients also display significant depression. Therefore, it is important initially to assess each patient for depression.

Treatment Strategies

Contingency contracting has been found very effective in helping the anorexic patient to gain weight (Brady & Rieger, 1972). Initially, obtaining cooperation from the patient and the family is important. The voluntary aspect of the contract should be emphasized. If the patient's weight is not medically dangerous, an outpatient contract can be attempted. In negotiating a contract, a goal weight

Table 1-1 Eating Attitudes Test

Please place an (X) under the column which applies best to each of the numbered statements. All of the results will be *strictly* confidential. Most of the questions directly relate to food or eating, although other types of questions have been included. Please answer each question carefully. Thank you.

Always	Very often	Often	Sometimes	Rarely	Never	Statement
( )	( )	( )	( )	( )	(X)†	1. Like eating with other people.
(X)	( )	( )	( )	( )	( )	2. Prepare foods for others but do not eat what I cook.
(X)	( )	( )	( )	( )	( )	3. Become anxious prior to eating.
(X)	( )	( )	( )	( )	( )	4. Am terrified about being overweight.
(X)	( )	( )	( )	( )	( )	5. Avoid eating when I am hungry.
(X)	( )	( )	( )	( )	( )	6. Find myself preoccupied with food.
(X)	( )	( )	( )	( )	( )	7. Have gone on eating binges where I feel that I may not be able to stop.
(X)	( )	( )	( )	( )	( )	8. Cut my food into small pieces.
(X)	( )	( )	( )	( )	( )	9. Aware of the calorie content of foods that I eat.
(X)	( )	( )	( )	( )	( )	10. Particularly avoid foods with a high carbohydrate content (e.g. bread, potatoes, rice, etc.).
(X)	( )	( )	( )	( )	( )	11. Feel bloated after meals.
(X)	( )	( )	( )	( )	( )	12. Feel that others would prefer if I ate more.
(X)	( )	( )	( )	( )	( )	13. **Vomit after I have eaten.
(X)	( )	( )	( )	( )	( )	14. Feel extremely guilty after eating.
(X)	( )	( )	( )	( )	( )	15. **Am preoccupied with a desire to be thinner.
(X)	( )	( )	( )	( )	( )	16. Exercise strenuously to burn off calories.
(X)	( )	( )	( )	( )	( )	17. **Weigh myself several times a day.
( )	( )	( )	( )	( )	(X)	18. ‡Like my clothes to fit tightly.
( )	( )	( )	( )	( )	(X)	19. Enjoy eating meat.
(X)	( )	( )	( )	( )	( )	20. Wake up early in the morning.
(X)	( )	( )	( )	( )	( )	21. Eat the same foods day after day.
(X)	( )	( )	( )	( )	( )	22. Think about burning up calories when I exercise.
( )	( )	( )	( )	( )	(X)	23. Have regular menstrual periods.
(X)	( )	( )	( )	( )	( )	24. Other people think that I am too thin.
(X)	( )	( )	( )	( )	( )	25. Am preoccupied with the thought of having fat on my body.
(X)	( )	( )	( )	( )	( )	26. Take longer than others to eat my meals.
( )	( )	( )	( )	( )	( )	27. Enjoy eating at restaurants.
(X)	( )	( )	( )	( )	( )	28. **Take laxatives.
(X)	( )	( )	( )	( )	( )	29. Avoid foods with sugar in them.
(X)	( )	( )	( )	( )	( )	30. Eat diet foods.
(X)	( )	( )	( )	( )	( )	31. Feel that food controls my life.
(X)	( )	( )	( )	( )	( )	32. Display self control around food.
(X)	( )	( )	( )	( )	( )	33. Feel that others pressure me to eat.
(X)	( )	( )	( )	( )	( )	34. Give too much time and thought to food.
(X)	( )	( )	( )	( )	( )	35. *Suffer from constipation.
(X)	( )	( )	( )	( )	( )	36. Feel uncomfortable after eating sweets.
(X)	( )	( )	( )	( )	( )	37. Engage in dieting behaviour.
(X)	( )	( )	( )	( )	( )	38. Like my stomach to be empty.
( )	( )	( )	( )	( )	(X)	39. Enjoy trying new rich foods.
(X)	( )	( )	( )	( )	( )	40. Have the impulse to vomit after meals.

(Garner and Garfinkel, 1979; p.278)

Table 1-2

ANOREXIC BEHAVIOR SCALE (22 ITEMS)

Respond YES, NO, or ? to the following items.

(a) Resistance to Eating

1. **Delays as much as possible before coming to the dining table.**
2. **Shows obvious signs of tension at meal times.**
3. **Shows increased hostility at meal times (towards nurses or food).**
4. **Begins by cutting up food into small pieces.**
5. **Complains that there is too much food or that it's too rich.**
6. **Exhibits extreme "food faddiness."**
7. **Bargains over food (e.g. "I'll eat X if I don't have to eat Y").**
8. **Picks at food (e.g. eating inside but leaving outside of potatoes, piecrusts, etc.).**

(b) Disposing of Food

9. **Vomits after meals.**
10. **Conceals food in serviettes, pockets, handbags and clothing.**
11. **Disposes of food out of windows, into dustbins, down sinks and toilets.**
12. **Conceals food in own room (e.g., in cupboards, drawers, flower vases, etc.).**
13. **Crumbles cakes into their wrapping paper.**
14. **Rubs food into clothes or spills liquids over own clothes.**
15. **Drops odd bits of food on the floor, e.g., peas.**
16. **Makes frequent use of purgatives or attempts to use purgatives.**

(c) Activity

17. **Stands as much as possible rather than sits.**
18. **Walks or runs about whenever possible.**
19. **Is as active and as industrious as possible (e.g., clearing tables, cleaning own room, etc.).**
20. **Chooses the more strenuous activity when given the choice (e.g. table tennis rather than watching television).**
21. **Makes unnecessary journeys for extra exercise.**
22. **Does physical exercises whenever possible (e.g., press-ups, etc.).**

(Slade, 1973; p. 85)

should be addressed. The goal weight can be the ideal weight for the patient, easily obtained from the life insurance tables of ideal weight, or it can be the patient's premorbid weight. It is suggested that the goal weight should be no lower than 90% of the ideal weight. It is also helpful to set an upper limit on the patient's weight since most anorexic patients are concerned about becoming obese. There is evidence that anorexic patients may continue to gain weight if there is no upper limit on the contract (Mavissakalian, 1982). Also include in the contract an agreement that the patient will be weighed daily, under standard conditions, and that the weight be graphed and posted in a conspicuous place in the patient's room. The recording or graphing of calories consumed may also add to the power of the informational feedback component (Agras, Barlow, Chapin, Abel, & Leitenberg, 1974). For patients unwilling to record calories, the number of mouthfuls eaten can be used as a substitute. Miller and Hebber (1979) successfully used the self-monitoring of bites of food as a negative reinforcer in treating an anorexic geriatric patient.

The contract should contain an agreement that the patient gain weight. Although many programs have used .5-pound weight gain per day criteria, it may be easier to shape the patient's behavior by starting with a .25-pound per day weight gain and eventually increasing to .5 pound per day. Initially, some medical problems may arise from rapid refeeding. To prevent a sporadic pattern of weight gain, it may be necessary to reinforce the patient for an increase in weight from the previously measured highest weight. A daily reward based on the information obtained during the assessment should be made contingent on the weight gain. The patient should be free to eat what she wants, and no attention should be given to her eating. The only exception to this is that a time limit should be set on each meal. If the patient maintains weight, or loses weight, it should be made clear that she will not have access to the rewards for that day. Bonus rewards, tied to specific weight goals, can also be incorporated into the contract.

Another important element of the contract is a statement that a maintenance contract will be negotiated when the patient reaches the goal weight. There should also be "critical" weights included in the contracts. For inpatients the critical weight, determined by a physician, is the point at which the contract is discontinued and the patient is too thin. For outpatients, the critical weight is the point at which the patient agrees to be rehospitalized.

A one- to two-week trial period for the contract is needed. If the patient does not gain weight during this period, the first consideration is to reevaluate the reinforcers chosen. A sample contingency contract is shown in Table 1-3.

Mavissakalian (1982) describes a typical in-patient contract as follows:

> **The treatment...utilized the following three sets of reinforcement contingencies. The first was an immediate reinforcement of appropriate eating behavior which meant that the patient, after the completion of an appropriate meal, could spend an hour outside of her room and engage in whatever activity she chose on the unit. Thus, she had the opportunity to earn a maximum of 3 hours per day outside her room.**
>
> **It is important to emphasize that a completed meal consisted of eating all that was presented to her within a 30-minute period. . . .**
>
> **The daily caloric presentation initially was 2000 calories which was raised to 3000 calories per day on the 20th day of treatment. . . .**

Table 1-3

Sample Contingency Contract

WEIGHT GAIN TREATMENT PLAN

The following plan is effective as of _________.

1. The goal of the following program is to achieve a minimum weight of __lbs. and a maximum weight of __ lbs. I agree to maintain that weight for two weeks before discharge. There will be four spot checks during the final two-week period. If I fall below 2 lbs. of the goal weight, the two-week period will be restarted following the reaching of the goal weight.

2. Each day I will be weighed by nursing staff at approximately the same time, before breakfast, dressed in sleepware. I will be told my weight by the nursing staff, and I agree to record this weight on a graph in my room.

3. I also agree to record the number of calories I eat per day and the number of mouthfuls I eat per day on separate graphs in my room.

4. If I gain _ lb. per day, above the previously highest recorded weight, I will receive the following each day (fill in reward).

5. Each day that I gain no weight or lose weight, I agree to (fill in response cost)

6. If I achieve the following weights, I will receive (fill in bonus reward).

7. I also agree that staff agreement to changes in the contents of this plan can only be made by ___________.

8. I agree that on days my weight is recorded as less than __ lbs., I will receive tube feedings, each consisting of __ calories of liquid nourishment.

9. I agree to negotiate a follow-up contract prior to discharge.

10. Failure to cooperate with the above plan may result in my discharge from the hospital.

The second set of reinforcements were of an intermediate nature and were contingently applied when the patient completed all three meals and met the minimal requirement of weight gain the next morning. The criterion for reinforcing daily weight gain was that the weight of that day should exceed the mean of the

> **weight of the previous two days. The reinforcement consisted of her spending the entire day out of her hospital room.**
>
> **Finally, the third set of reinforcements were rather delayed since they were contingent on reaching a certain level of weight and determined the general level of activity and increasing freedom from hospital restrictions, i.e., ground privileges, passes and discharge from the hospital. As a note, the first and second sets of reinforcement contingencies remained operative to the very last day of her hospitalization which meant that even though the patient had reached a certain weight which permitted her to spend her days away from the hospital, if she did not complete an observable meal (breakfast and dinner which took place in the hospital) and/or did not meet the minimum required increase in daily weight, she became restricted to her room for that day and the first set of contingencies applied for that day. [p. 28]**

Some in-patient programs have chosen to use access from a very restricted environment as a reinforcer. In this treatment, the patient is initially placed in a room containing only essential furniture. She would remain in bed during the day, including meal times. After the meals are served in the patient's room, the food should be left with the patient for a set amount of time (30 to 45 minutes), even if the patient does not eat. One program provides the patient with her own refrigerator and scales in the room. In addition to individual rewards, some standard rewards have usually proven successful. These include phone privileges, visiting privileges, access to activities, and passes off the ward. Neumann and Gaoni (1975) have used preferred food as a reinforcer.

Other in-patient programs start with the more restricted program, progress to a more individual reward program, and then move to a program where the patient has more self-control and responsibility. This may involve staff weighings every other day, and eventually once a week. However, the patient would be free to take the responsibility to weigh herself on the days the staff does not weigh her.

The anorexic patient tends to eat more when presented with larger portions of food (Elkin, Hersen, Eisler, & Williams, 1973; Agras et al., 1974). Therefore, the patient should be served double portions at all meals. If rapid refeeding is a concern, it is suggested that the amount of calories offered to the patient be determined by a food nomogram (see, for example Boothby and Berkson food nomogram, Mayo Clinic, 1951).

Halmi, Powers, and Cunningham (1975) suggest that during the first week of the program the patient be offered 125% of the basal requirements, 150% the second week, and 200% the third week. The fourth week the patient is served three regular diet meals. Follow-up contracts can include random telephone scheduling of appointments for weighing.

After the patient has reached the goal weight, the focus of a contingency contract should shift to weight maintenance. Patients should be encouraged to maintain their weight within a 3- to 5-pound range rather than at a specific weight. Maintenance should include the return of more control to the patient and the fading of therapist contact. The use of significant others to maintain a contract can be a good intermediate step if both parties agree. The granting of rewards for maintaining weight can be switched from being provided by others to a self-reward program. Contingencies can be provided for any recorded weight that is outside of either end of the agreed-upon weight range. Weight and calorie graphings should continue. A rehospitalization weight should be included in a maintenance contract.

In addition to a weight gain program, there are other adjunctive techniques that are helpful with anorexics. Cognitive behavioral techniques can be useful in dealing with the anorexic's distorted thoughts. Garner and Bemis (1982) suggest some possible ways to utilize cognitive behavioral therapy with anorexics:

1) Encoure the patient to look at the practical implications of her belief in thinness.

2) Educate the patient about the symptoms, risk, and course of anorexia nervosa.

3) Use cognitive techniques of operationalizing beliefs, decentering, "what if," evaluating automatic thoughts, hypothesis testing, and modifying basic assumptions.

4) Reinterpretation of body image misperceptions.

Some programs have incorporated systematic desensitization to deal with food phobias, fear of eating with other people, a fear of becoming obese, and sexual fears. Schnurer, Rubin, and Roy (1973) used two hierarchies for systematic desensitization treatment with one patient. One hierarchy dealt with the patient's perceived changes in appearance with increased weight, and the second hierarchy dealt with the anxiety associated with eating specific foods.

Assertion training and social skills training have been used to get the anorexic patient to express feelings directly and to improve interpersonal communication. However, these treatments alone may not have any effect on the anorexic's weight (Pillay & Crisp, 1981).

If bulimic behaviors are also present, some of the techniques discussed in the chapter on bulimia may have to be implemented. (See Chapter 6.)

Another helpful adjunct to an operant program is to attempt to change some of the family interactions with the anorexic patient. For the patient who lives at home, Poole, Sanson-Fischer, and Young (1978) have suggested the following guidelines for their families:

1) avoid any reinforcement of invalid behavior or complaints;

2) do not make an issue of eating;

3) reinforce maintenance of the patient's weight by verbal reinforcement;

4) do not prepare any special diet for the patient;

5) do not weigh the patient at home;

6) discuss only pleasant topics at meal times; and

7) encourage the patient to dine out with other people under enjoyable conditions.

It may also be useful for the clinician to attend a family meal to observe the interaction and communication patterns and, if necessary, teach the family how to eat together without a power struggle.

For patients who resist the operant program, a seemingly paradoxical intention orientation may be helpful. Hsu and Lieberman (1982) suggest that patients be told to continue to be anorexic. They then are told what reinforcement they are obtaining from the disorder. Finally, they are told that they can disagree with the therapist's explanation and can continue to be seen in therapy.

Rosen (1980) deals with the modification of secretive and ritualized eating behavior in anorexics with another paradoxical method. The patients are instructed to only eat in their maladaptive style. They can only eat foods that are "secretly obtained" or "hidden." The eating has to be done alone. If the patient does not follow the agreement, or if the patient's weight decreases, they are to be hospitalized immediately. The patient can return to normal eating only after totally rejecting the maladaptive eating behavior. This technique can work very rapidly (often in one to three days) to change the maladaptive eating behavior.

For More Information

Agras, S., & Werne, J. (1979). Behavior therapy in anorexia nervosa: A data-based approach to the question. In J. Brady & H. Brodie (Eds.), *Controversy in psychiatry,* (pp. 655-673). Philadelphia: W.B. Saunders Co.

This chapter reviews the behavioral studies of anorexia. Immediate and long-term outcomes are discussed. Specific suggestions for in-patient treatment are included. The book can be obtained from W.B. Saunders Co., W. Washington Square, Philadelphia, PA 19105.

Bemis, K. (1978). Current approaches to the etiology and treatment of the anorexia nervosa. *Psychological Bulletin, 85*, 593-617.

A general review article covering incidence, clinical picture, family background, premorbid characteristics, precipitating factors, outcome, and the therapeutic approaches of psychodynamics, family interaction, and medical and behavioral treatments. The article can be obtained from Kelly M. Bemis, Department of Psychology, University of Minnesota, Elliott Hall, 75 East River Road, Minneapolis, Minnesota 55455.

Garner, D., & Bemis, K. (1982). A cognitive behavioral approach to anorexia nervosa. *Cognitive Therapy and Research, 6*, 123-150.

An excellent description of cognitive behavioral techniques that can be applied to the anorexic patient. There is also a good theoretical discussion of the development of anorexia nervosa. The article can be obtained from David Garner, Ph.D., Clark Institute of Psychiatry, 250 College Street, Toronto, Canada M5TIR8.

References

Agras, S., Barlow, D., Chapen, H., Abel, G., & Leitenberg, H. (1974). Behavior modification of anorexia nervosa, *Archives of General Psychiatry, 30*, 270-286.

Brady, J., & Rieger, W. (1975). Behavioral treatment of anorexia nervosa. In T. Thompson & W. Dockens (Eds.), *Applications of behavior modification* (pp. 45-63). New York: Academic Press.

Cautela, J., & Castenbaum, R. (1967). Reinforcement survey schedule for use in therapy, training and research. *Psychological Reports, 29*, 1115-1130.

Elkin, T., Hersen, M., Eisler, R., & Williams, J. (1973). Modification of caloric intake in anorexia nervosa: An experimental analysis. *Psychological Reports, 32*, 75-78.

Garner, D., & Bemis, K. (1982). A cognitive behavioral approach to anorexia nervosa. *Cognitive Theory and Research, 6*, 123-150.

Garner, D., & Garfinkel, P. (1979). The Eating Attitudes Test: An index of the symptoms of anorexia nervosa. *Psychological Medicine, 9*, 273-279.

Halmi, K., Powers, P., & Cunningham, S. (1975). Treatment of anorexia nervosa with behavior modification. *Archives of General Psychiatry, 32*, 93-96.

Hsu, L., & Lieberman, S. (1982). Paradoxical intention in the treatment of chronic anorexia nervosa. *American Journal of Psychiatry, 139*, 650-653.

Mavissakalian, M. (1982). Anorexia nervosa treated with response prevention and prolonged exposure. *Behavior Research and Therapy, 20*, 27-31.

Mayo Clinic (1951). Boothby and Berkson food nomogram. *Postgraduate Medicine, 9*, 109.

Milberg, W., & Hebber, N. (1979). Termination of self-monitoring as a negative reinforcer to increase weight gain in a 77 year-old anorexic male. *The Behavior Therapist, 2*, 21-22.

Neumann, M., & Gaoni, B. (1975). Preferred food as the reinforcing agent in a case of anorexia nervosa. *Journal of Behavior Therapy and Experimental Psychiatry, 6*, 331-333.

Pillay, M., & Crisp, A. (1981). The impact of social skills training within an established in-patient treatment programme for anorexia nervosa. *British Journal of Psychiatry, 139*, 533-539.

Poole, A., Samson-Fischer, R., & Young, P. (1978). A behavioral programme for the management of anorexia nervosa. *Australian and New Zealand Journal of Psychiatry, 12*, 49-53.

Rosen, L. (1980). Modification of secretive or ritualized eating behavior in anorexia nervosa. *Journal of Behavior Therapy and Experimental Psychiatry, 11*, 101-104.

Schnurer, A., & Rubin, R. (1973). Systematic desensitization of anorexia nervosa seen as a weight phobia. *Journal of Behavior Therapy and Experimental Psychiatry, 11*, 101-104.

Slade, P. (1973). A short anorexic behavior scale. *British Journal of Psychiatry, 122*, 83-85.

See Also

Chapter 6. Bulimia

2 Anxiety —Stressful Medical Procedures

Assessment Strategies

The prospect of many medical procedures (e.g., endoscopy or cardiac catheterization) can create significant anxiety. The patient's anxiety rating may be obtained prior to, during, and after the procedure. Wilson (1981) describes a mood rating schedule used with elective surgery patients as follows:

> **Patients were asked to indicate how much they felt (on a four-point scale ranging from "not at all"to "very much"): afraid, jittery, uneasy, incapable, unable, helpless, grouchy, irritated, annoyed, alert, energetic, active, good, cheerful, satisfied. All 15 adjectives were summed to form an index of mood, with negative moods numerically reversed. [p. 84]**

Anxiety inventories, such as the State-Trait Anxiety Inventory, may be used to supplement these pain ratings. A Depression-Sensitization Scale (Epstein & Fenz, 1967) may also be helpful in selecting appropriate treatment strategies.

Personality variables may also be used as indices of degree of stress experienced in response to a medical procedure. Wilson (1981) measured preoperative fear, level of denial, and level of aggressiveness. Preoperative fear was rated on a seven-point Likert scale by having the patient provide ratings for the following three questions: "Are you worried about your operation?" "Are you worried about your illness?" "Are you worried about going under anesthesia?" (Wilson, 1981; p. 85). Level of denial was measured on a five-point scale by having the patient provide ratings for the following three questions:

> **"Most things will generally turn out all right if you just leave them alone." . . . "Worrying ahead of time about bad things that might happen makes it easier for me to handle them later on." . . . "It's best not to think about the future when something unpleasant is going to happen." [Wilson, 1981, p. 85]**
>
> **Level of aggressiveness was assessed by having the patient take a short form of the Defense Mechanism Inventory. Patients responded to hypothetical situations, such as being splashed with mud by a passing bus, by selecting from among five behaviors that vary in the extent to which anger or aggressive behavior is directly expressed. A single aggressiveness score was calculated by combining the five subscales of the DMI (Protection plus Turning against object; Reversal; Turning against self; Principalization). [Wilson, 1981; pp. 85-86]**

Behavioral observation of the patient can be used to assess anxiety occurring during the procedure. Johnson, Morrissey, and Leventhal (1973) observed hand and arm movements and general restlessness exhibited by patients undergoing endoscopic examinations. Psychophysiological data on anxiety and distress, including pulse and heart-rate measures, can also be obtained.

Finally, several post-procedural indices of anxiety and distress can be used.

The patient's ambulation may be assessed by observation or by self-report. Length of hospital stay may also be employed. Wilson (1981) used a "recovery inventory" described as follows:

> **Patients were asked to rate their physical condition on six-point scales with the following categories: appetite, strength and energy, stomach condition, bowel condition, ability to urinate, ability to do things for themselves, ability to move around, and interest in what is going on around them. [p. 84]**

If the patient presents with injection phobia, the strength of the fear can be measured by using a Behavioral Approach Test (BAT) for injection phobias (see Table 2-1).

The patient can record each item on the hierarchy that is either upsetting in imagination or in vivo. Then, the patient can determine his Subjective Units of Disturbance (SUDS) for those items on a 100-point scale, 0 indicating no anxiety, 100 indicating the most anxiety. The SUDS rating can be used as a pre-assessment/post-assessment measure, or as a daily record during treatment intervention.

Table 2-1

BEHAVIORAL APPROACH TEST AND HIERARCHY FOR SYSTEMATIC DESENSITIZATION OF INJECTION PHOBIA

18	Receiving injection by physician
17	Syringe, shield off, held by Th and darted quickly to S's arm
16	Syringe, shield on, held by Th and darted quickly to S's arm
15	Syringe, shield off, held by S and darted quickly to Th's arm
14	Syringe, shield on, held by S and darted quickly to Th's arm
13	Syringe, shield off, held by Th and touched to S's arm
12	Syringe, shield on, held by Th and touched to S's arm
11	Syringe, shield off, held by S and touched to her own arm
10	Syringe, shield on, held by S and touched to her own arm
9	Syringe, shield off, held by S and touched to Th's arm
8	Syringe, shield on, held by S and touched to Th's arm
7	Syringe is placed leaning against S's arm, shield off
6	Syringe is placed leaning against S's arm, shield on
5	Being prepared for an injection (sleeve up, rubbed with swab)
4	Handling syringe with shield off
3	Handling syringe with shield on
2	Viewing syringe on table with shield off the needle
1	Viewing hypodermic syringe on table with shield on the needle

[Nimmer and Kapp, 1974; p. 258]

S denotes subject; Th denotes therapist.

Treatment Strategies

Information may be helpful in reducing anxiety in some patients. Shipley, Butt, Horwitz, and Farbry (1978) found that "sensitizers" benefit from extensive preparation for stressful medical procedures while "repressors" fare best when left alone.

Sensory information has been found to be more effective than procedural information (Fuller, Endress, & Johnson, 1978; Johnson & Leventhal, 1974). Procedural information describes the medical procedure itself, while sensory information describes what the patient will experience. Shipley (1982) describes a typical sensory information procedure as follows:

> **As you slowly wake up in the recovery room, you will feel confused, drowsy, and forgetful for a while; you may not know where you are or what time of the day it is. What you see and hear will be fuzzy for a while and you may hear talking or possibly groaning in the distance or coming from yourself. As you awaken, you may notice some details of the recovery room such as. . . . The incision on the right side of your abdomen will be tender and sensitive; you may feel pressure, pulling, smarting, or painful burning sensations. These painful sensations may become sharp and seem to travel along the incision. This pain is quite normal and to be expected. You may also have a sore throat caused by drying of the throat and by irritation from a tube put down your throat to help you breathe while you were in surgery. To help make the pain tolerable, you will be getting medication. You will know when you get medication either by the feel of a shot or by the nurse telling you she has put medication in the intravenous tube in your vein.**
>
> **You may notice nurses checking your pulse and blood pressure about every 15 minutes, and taking your temperature occasionally. As you come awake, the recovery room nurses will encourage you to turn from side to side, to take deep breaths, and to cough to remove material that may have accumulated in your lungs. It will be somewhat painful for you to breathe deeply and cough; these activities may increase the pressure, pulling, and smarting sensations mentioned earlier. However, deep breathing and coughing are necessary to avoid fever and pneumonia. [pp. 71-72]**

Viewing a videotape of the procedure can also reduce anxiety (Shipley, 1978). Additionally, Shipley et al. (1978) found that viewing the videotape three times reduced the patient's anxiety more than viewing the videotape only once.

Dziurbejko and Larkin (1978) found that providing the information to the patient and the family together was more effective than providing information only to the patient.

Wilson (1981) employed muscle relaxation training with elective surgery patients. He found that less frightened patients benefited more from relaxation than did very frightened patients. Relaxation training has been successfully used in combination with an information procedure (Fuller et al., 1978).

Egbert, Battit, Welch, and Bartlett (1964) found that relaxation combined with information increased the patient's comfort after the medical procedure.

A cognitive-behavioral intervention has also been found to be effective in reducing anxiety in patients scheduled to undergo cardiac catheterization the following day (Kendall et al., 1979). They describe the procedure as follows:

> **Patients in this group received individual training in the discrimination of anxiety-producing cues and in the application of their own individual and personal coping strategies in response to such cues. The training was accomplished in well-defined**

> stages. Patients were initially informed that the training procedure was designed to help them feel less anxious and more comfortable with the impending catheterization. Relaxation and the reduction of anxiety were described as important components in the process of being a better patient. Stress was explained as a response that everyone experiences and copes with in some way. The therapist then self-disclosed some source of real stress in his or her own life along with the strategy he or she had employed to reduce the experienced stress. Thus, patients received a "coping" model who initially self-disclosed the fears and subsequently the methods for overcoming them.... Similar self-disclosure regarding previous stress and stress-related cues was then elicited from the patient. At this point, the therapist had several examples of stress reduction strategies that the patient had disclosed as being useful in the past and proceded to discuss these in relation to the cues that the patient identified as elicitors of anxiety. For example, if the patient identified the "machinery" of the hospital as being "beyond" understanding and therefore ominous, the therapist would model cognitive coping skills such as "science has come such a long way to be able to have and use all this expensive equipment and the doctors are very skilled in their use." The patient was then instructed to use his anxiety-producing cues as prompts for the application of his cognitive coping skills and to reassure himself of his ability to relax and cope with stress as he experienced decreased arousal. The therapist conducted behavioral rehearsal with the patient concerning the entire process of discriminating anxiety-related cues, applying cognitive coping skills, and labeling the experience as an example of self-effacious coping. [p. 51]

Langer, Janis, and Wolfer (1975) successfully employed a procedure in which patients were instructed in cognitive reappraisal of surgery as a stressful event. Patients used selective attention to focus on the positive factors (e.g., the hospital stay served as a period of rest) and to exclude the negative factors of the surgery.

Taylor, Ferguson, and Wermuth (1977) found that participant modeling was an effective procedure in treating anxiety in patients with an injection phobia. They describe the procedure as follows:

> The treating resident explained the procedure briefly to the patient, told him it would take approximately 1 hr and that he would be asked to touch and experiment with some of the intravenous equipment, syringes and needles. He was told that after this hour he would feel more comfortable with these items and blood-drawing, and that the treatment would culminate with the therapist drawing his blood.... He brought a tray with packaged tubing, syringes, tape, local anaesthetics, gauze, alcohol swabs, needles, etc., into the treatment room and asked the patient if he was comfortable with the instrument-filled tray in the room. (If the patient had reported discomfort, the therapist would have taken the tray out of the room and introduced one item at a time.) The therapist then picked up the packaged materials one at a time, identified them, and handed them to the patient, each time pausing until the patient felt comfortable touching the packages. The patient was asked to remove the articles from the packages, which he did slowly. He was then asked to examine progressively larger covered needles. When the patient was able to accomplish these tasks comfortably, the therapist removed the cover from a needle and handed it to the patient. This was done with progressively larger sized needles. When the patient no longer felt anxious holding a syringe with a bared needle, the therapist touched the needle to his own skin. The patient was able to copy this action and proceeded to rub the needle up and down his arm. Then the therapist put a needle on a second syringe and filled it with procaine. The patient held the medication-filled syringe until he felt at ease. The experimenter then injected procaine into an orange and asked the patient to copy his actions, which

he did several times without reporting any fear. He was able to use progressively larger needles to inject the orange. Then the experimenter attached a tuberculin-sized needle to a syringe and lightly stroked the back of his arm and then stuck it in the back of his arm. The patient was then asked to, and was able to have this done to him. The experimenter then put a larger needle on the syringe and said that he was going to draw blood. He asked the patient to watch as he applied a tourniquet and stuck the needle into the patient's arm to draw blood. The patient complained that he didn't like the procedure and looked away. The therapist gently coaxed him to look at the needle in his arm which the patient was able to do. Approximately 1 hr. was needed for the entire procedure. [p. 30]

Imagery has been used with success in the reduction of anxiety associated with stressful medical procedures. Cohn, Kron, and Brady (1976) taught a patient to use anger induction via imagery to treat blood-illness-injury phobia. Cohn et al. (1976) describe the procedure as follows:

...the patient was shown four stimulus pictures projected on a screen at approximately one-half size using a carousel 35-mm slide projector. Three of the slides were obtained from the Office of The Medical Examiner and depicted mutilated bodies. . . . An alternate technique was attempted, that of having the patient replace his fearful response to the phobic stimulus with an alternate and mutually exclusive emotion, that of anger. Four situations associated with especially angry feelings were identified by the patient: a) his father's criticisms of the patient's life style; b) an argument which had occurred during his draft induction; c) a recent fight with his wife; and d) hostile feelings toward his graduate school advisor. The therapist attempted to help the patient by role-playing the antagonist while the patient was simultaneously exposed to the phobic slide. [pp. 66-67]

Systematic desensitization has been an effective procedure in treating anxiety related to medical procedures and anxiety resulting from blood or injection phobias. Elmore, Wildman, and Westefeld (1980) describe the use of systematic desensitizationwith a blood phobic patient as follows:

Approximately five sessions of systematic desensitization . . . were conducted. The hierarchy in Table 1 was part of the standard treatment. The lowest five scenes on the hierarchy were covered prior to the switch to *in vivo* procedures.

Table 1
ANXIETY HIERARCHY FOR SYSTEMATIC DESENSITIZATION SESSIONS

SUDS	Scene
100	Someone covered with blood, such as a person lying on the side of the road after an automobile accident
90	Blood gushing from a cut as happened the summer of the 6th grade when a friend fell and cut his arm
80	Talking about surgery, as happened in a high school biology class
70	Waiting to have a blood sample taken

60	**Having a blood sample taken**
50	**Visiting a blood bank without giving or seeing blood**
40	**An empty blood bag**
30	**Advertisement for blood giving**
20	**Accidental prick of right finger**
10	**Red construction paper**
0	**Summer afternoon under a tree at home**

> **. . . Slides taken from anatomical and surgical texts were introduced as phobic stimuli in the relaxation sessions. . . . The patient now began questioning the slides' relevance, pointing out that he . . . had no plans to become a physician. He suggested slides made of himself moving through the process of giving blood at a local Red Cross Donor Center. He felt that the ability to give blood comfortably would be a realistic goal incompatible with his phobia . . . The patient then took the slides home and used them in self-conducted desensitization sessions. This auto-desensitization was carried out two to three times per week over an 8-week period. Towards the end of this period, the patient began to introduce into the sessions objects associated with medical procedures and blood. Objects used were a thermometer, a glass tube, a blood-pressure apparatus and a hypodermic needle. . . Following the at-home desensitization sessions, it was decided to conduct an *in vivo* test of the effectiveness of the treatment. [p. 278]**

In the case of injection phobia, for some patients it is possible to eradicate the phobia by correcting misconceptions about injection injuries. If this is not successful at eliminating the phobia, imagined or *in vivo* systematic desensitization may be used with hierarchy described in Table 1.

In the *in vivo* desensitization, it would be helpful to include medicinal odors, such as ether or alcohol, since they often trigger fear responses. Also, the use of modeling, live or on film, would give the patient the opportunity to watch appropriate non-phobic reactions to injections.

For More Information

Anderson, K., and Masur, F. (1983). Psychological preparation for invasive medical and dental procedures. *Journal of Behavioral Medicine, 6*, 1-40.

This article reviews the research that has been done on informative approaches in preparing patients for invasive medical and dental procedures. Then the psychotherapeutic approaches of modeling, relaxation, systematic desensitization, and behavior management are reviewed. The cognitive-behavioral approaches are also reviewed. Studies with both adults and children are included. A discussion of methodological problems, legal-ethical considerations, and cost effectiveness is also included. The article can be obtained from Dr. Frank Masur, 6005 Park Avenue, Suite 903, Memphis, TN 38119.

Schultheis, K., Peterson, L., & Selby, V. (1987). Preparation for stressful medical procedures and person and treatment interactions. *Clinical Psychology Review, 7*, 329-352.

This article reviews the treatment approaches of procedural information, sensory information, coping instructions, and modelling. The influence on the treatment of person characteristics such as gender, locus of control, coping styles, and test anxiety is then discussed. The article can be obtained from Karen Schultheis, VAMC, 116B, 4500 South Lancaster, Dallas, TX 75216.

Shipley, R. (1982). Behavioral management of acute anxiety and pain of stressful medical procedures. In P. Boudewyns and F. Keefe (Eds.), *Behavioral medicine in general medicine practice*. Reading, Mass.: Addison-Wesley.

This chapter is an excellent review of all the procedures available. It includes informational approaches, behavioral coping strategies, and cognitive approaches. A detailed example of the cognitive treatment is included. The book can be obtained from Addison-Wesley Publishing Co., 1 Jacob Way, Reading, Mass. 01867.

References

Cohn, C., Kron, R., & Brady, J. (1978). A case of blood-illness-injury phobia treated behaviorally.. *The Journal of Nervous and Mental Disease, 162*, 65-68.

Dziurbejko, M., & Larkin, J., (1978). Including the family in pre-operative teaching. *American Journal of Nursing*, 1892-1894.

Egbert, L., Battit, G., Welch, C., & Bartlett, M. (1964). Reduction of post-operative pain by encouragement and instruction. *New England Journal of Medicine, 270*, 825-827.

Elmore, R., Wildman, R., & Westfeld, J. (1980). The use of systematic desensitization in the treatment of blood phobia. *Journal of Behavior Therapy and Experimental Psychiatry, 11*, 277-279.

Epstein, S., & Fenz, W. (1967). The detection of areas of emotional stress through variations in perceptual threshold and physiological arousal. *Journal of Experimental Research in Personality, 2*, 191-199.

Fuller, S., Endress, P., & Johnson, J. (1978). The effects of cognitive and behavioral control on coping with an adversive health examination. *Journal of Human Stress*, 18-25.

Johnson, J., & Leventhal, H., (1974). Effects of accurate expectations and behavioral instructions on reactions during a noxious medical examination. *Journal of Personality and Social Psychology, 5*, 710-178.

Johnson, J., Morrissey, J., & Leventhal, H. (1973). Psychological preparation for an endoscopic examination. *Gastrointestinal Endoscopy, 19*, 180-182.

Kendall, P., Williams, L., Pechacek, T., Graham, L., Shisslak, C., & Herzoff, N., (1979). Cognitive-behavioral and patient educational interventions in cardiac catheterization procedures: The Palo Alto medical psychology project. *Journal of Consulting and Clinical Psychology, 47*, 49-58.

Langer, E., Janis, I., & Wolfer, J. (1975). Reduction of psychological stress in surgical patients. *Journal of Experimental Social Psychology, 11*, 155-165.

Nimmer, W., & Kapp, R. (1974). A multiple impact program for the treatment of injection phobias. *Journal of Behavior Therapy and Experimental Psychiatry, 5*, 257-258.

Shipley, R. (1982). Behavioral managment of acute anxiety and pain of stressful medical procedures. In P. Boudewyns and F. Keefe (Eds.) *Behavioral medicine in general medicine practice* (pp. 68-93). Reading, MA: Addison-Wesley.

Shipley, R., Butt, J., Horwitz, B., & Farbry, J. (1978). Preparation for a stressful medical procedure: effect of amount of stimulus pre-exposure and coping style. *Journal of Consulting and Clinical Psychology, 46*, 499-507.

Taylor, C., Ferguson, J., & Wermuth, B. (1977). Simple techniques to treat medical phobias. *Postgraduate Medical Journal, 53*, 28-32.

Wilson, J. (1981). Behavioral preparation of surgery: Benefit or harm? *Journal of Behavioral Medicine, 4*, 79-102.

See Also

Chapter 29. Pain - Acute

3 Aphasia

Assessment Strategies

Aphasia is a term used to describe the acquired impairment of language processes. This impairment is a result of damage to areas of the brain implicated in language. Aphasia may occur in response to brain damage resulting from head trauma, cerebrovascular accidents, or a number of diseases. The aphasic patient may present one or more of the following symptoms: impairment in spoken language, written language, or writing; poor auditory comprehension; perseveration. A physical evaluation is necessary to determine the source and extent of damage.

In assessing degree of impairment, a base rate of responding should be established. This can be accomplished by asking the patient to respond to a standard set of questions (e.g., "Describe what you are wearing."). The patient's responses may be assessed for the number of sentences, words or phrases, unrecognizable utterances, disfluencies, and incidents of perseveration exhibited. There are several psychological test batteries that have been used to assess aphasia. Examples include the Minnesota Test for Differential Diagnosis of Aphasia (Schuell, 1965) and the Porch Index of Communication (Porch, 1967). A brief aphasia screening test has also been developed by Halstead and Wepman (1959).

In addition to language difficulty, the aphasic patient may present related disorders which can contribute to the difficulty in communication. These include apraxia, disarthria, and disrhythmia, among others. To determine locus and degree of disability, a neurological and/or neuropsychological examination is necessary.

The aphasic patient may experience anxiety as a result of the aphasia. Anxiety may play a role in exacerbating the language impairment. Furthermore, the patient may attempt to mitigate the anxiety by avoiding social situations in which the impairment is evidenced. Therefore, an evaluation of level of anxiety and accompanying patterns of social avoidance is often indicated.

Treatment Strategies

Operant conditioning has been used with success in the treatment of aphasic patients. Basic components of operant conditioning include shaping and differential reinforcement.

Programmed instruction (Holland, 1970) is an example of a structured language program which comprises elements of operant conditioning. Holland (1970) describes a typical programmed instruction as follows:

> **All of the programmed training began with a simple response already within the repertoire of a particular patient and moved toward more complex responses—either by requiring the patient to produce more words, by requiring the patient to make alternative selections among previously taught simple responses, or by using progressively more complex (or subtle) stimulus material (items), or by some combination or sequencing of all of these. In most cases, the programs were pre-**

> **pared on 3" x 5" index cards, if the items required the patient to read. Answers requiring writing were generally made on cards. Spoken items were sometimes tape-recorded but were most frequently simply presented by live voice from a previously written script. [p. 379]**
>
> **Group therapy incorporating the procedures of shaping and reinforcement has been employed with aphasic patients. One such example is Matrix Games (Holland, 1970), a program designed initially to develop verbal categorization skills in children. Matrix Games consists of a series of 3 x 3 or 4 x 4 picture matrices, each with a general theme and with relationships between pictures in its rows and columns. Typically, children name the pictures, and explore verbally the relationship between the grouped sets. The aphasia group used the pictures in this way, as naming and categorizing exercises. Since the pictures also lent themselves to such use, they were the basis for teaching plurality, subject-verb agreement, past tense, and simple syntactical ordering. [Holland, 1970, p. 385]**

Goodkin (1966) developed another treatment program based on operant conditioning that included the use of a token economy system in which blue poker chips were delivered contingent on correct responses and red poker chips were given contingent on incorrect responses. In addition, this program used the technique of modeling to reinforce the acquisition of the contingencies. Correct and incorrect responses were modeled by the experimenter, who self-administered the corresponding contingencies.

In cases in which anxiety has been clearly identified as a contributing factor in language difficulty, systematic desensitization has been implemented in the reduction of anxiety levels (Ince, 1968).

A modification of systematic desensitization has been combined with deep muscle relaxation and operant conditioning in treating aphasia and accompanying anxiety (Damon, Lesser, & Woods, 1979). The muscle relaxation was practiced at home with the assistance of the patient's significant other. The patient was encouraged to employ this technique in actual instances of anxiety. The modified systematic desensitization included construction of a hierarchy of anxiety-provoking situations with subsequent exposure to real-life situations. In addition, the patient received verbal reinforcement for successes and for attempts.

For More Information

Holland, A. (1970). Case studies in aphasia rehabilitation using programmed instruction. *Journal of Speech and Hearing Disorders, 35*, 377-390.

This article describes a technique for language rehabilitation for an aphasic population and reviews seven case records in which this technique was applied. The article can be obtained from Audrey Holland, University of Pittsburgh, Pittsburgh, PA 15213.

References

Damon, S., Lesser, R., & Woods, R. (1979). Behavioral treatment of social difficulties with an aphasic woman and a dysarthric man. *British Journal of Disorders of Communication, 14*, 31-38.

Goodkin, R. (1966). Case studies in behavioral research in rehabilitation. *Perceptual and Motor Skills, 23*, 171-182.

Goodkin, R. (1968). Use of concurrent response categories in evaluating talking behavior in aphasic patients. *Perceptual and Motor Skills, 26*, 1035-1040.

Halstead, W., & Wepman, J. (1959). The Halstead-Wepman Aphasia Screening Test. *Journal of Speech and Hearing Disorders, 14*, 9-15.

Ince, L. (1968). Desensitization with an aphasic patient. *Behavior Research and Therapy, 6*, 235-237.

Porch, B. (1967). *Porch Index of Communicative Ability*. Palo Alto, CA: Consulting Psychologists Press.

Schuell, H. (1965). *Differential diagnosis of aphasia with the Minnesota Test.* Minneapolis: University of Minnesota Press.

4 Asthma

Assessment Strategies

In 1975, Mathison described the symptoms of asthma:

> **To the patient, asthma means labored breathing accompanied by wheezing, a sense of chest constriction, and frequently coughing, gasping, and apprehension. To the physician, asthma should mean reversible obstruction of the bronchial airways caused by smooth muscle constriction, mucosal edema, and the retention of secretions with resultant symptoms and signs of respiratory insufficiency. [p. 524]**

A distinction is often made between extrinsic asthma in which there is an aggravation of symptoms after contact with an environmental allergen, such as dust, and intrinsic asthma where no allergen can be identified. Several different types of assessments may be useful in dealing with the presenting problem of asthma. There are two common physiological measurements that have been used: Peak Forced Expiratory Flow Rate (PEFR) and Forced Expiratory Volume, one second (FEV1). Knapp and Wells (1978) describe the procedures as follows: "Both measures require an apparatus (flow meter) into which the subject exhales with as much force as possible following an inspiration to maximum capacity. The PEFR is the rate of air out flow at the peak of the expiration curve, while FEV1 is the volume of air expired during the first second" (p. 105). Often three measurements are taken when using these procedures. Erskine and Schonell (1979) had their patients give a subjective severity rating of the asthma for each measurement of FEV1.

Several different self-report measures can also be used to assess asthma. These include: the number of attacks daily, the frequency of bronchometer use, medication use, and duration of bedtime coughing (using a tape recorder if necessary). Erskine and Schonell (1979) have developed daily and weekly symptom questionnaires (see Tables 4-1 and 4-2) for the patient to fill in during assessment and treatment.

In addition to the above measures, a behavioral diary that includes the precipitants of an attack may be useful. For many patients, anxiety, stress, or both may precipitate or exacerbate an attack. It is therefore necessary to include an assessment of general anxiety (e.g., State-Trait Anxiety Scale) or an assessment of a specific fear (e.g., the fear of an attack or the fear of dying).

Treatment Strategies

Relaxation training alone has had mixed results with asthma patients. Phillip, Wilde, and Day (1972) found that a modified Wolpe relaxation technique that emphasized breathing and abdominal muscles was effective in treating asthma patients after five sessions. However, Erskine and Schonell (1979) did not find a muscular or mental relaxation technique effective. Wilson, Honsberger, Child, and Novey (1975) successfully used transcendental meditation to treat asthma

Table 4-1

WEEKLY SYMPTOM QUESTIONNAIRE*

Indicate which of the following symptoms you have had during the past week. First, check the severity of the symptoms; then check the frequency of the symptoms. (See below.)

	Severity	Frequency
1. Panting	________	________
2. Numb	________	________
3. Mucous congestion	________	________
4. Cranky	________	________
5. Irritable	________	________
6. Hard to breathe	________	________
7. Headache	________	________
8. Edgy	________	________
9. Frightened	________	________
10. Short of breath	________	________
11. Chest congestion	________	________
12. Itchy lungs	________	________
13. Afraid of dying	________	________
14. Frustrated with things	________	________
15. Dizzy	________	________
16. Rapid breathing	________	________
17. Worn out	________	________
18. Panicky	________	________
19. Weak	________	________
20. Pins and needles feelings	________	________
21. Itchy throat	________	________
22. Wheezy	________	________
23. Worried about attack	________	________
24. Tingly in spots	________	________
25. Chest tightening	________	________
26. Scared	________	________
27. Shallow breathing	________	________
28. Choking	________	________
29. Fatigued	________	________
30. Chest filling up	________	________
31. Tense muscles	________	________
32. Short tempered	________	________
33. Worried	________	________
34. Anxious	________	________
35. Itchy skin	________	________
36. Nauseated	________	________
37. Coughing	________	________
38. No energy	________	________
39. Worried about self	________	________

SCALES

Severity	*Frequency*
E = Very severe	5 = All of the time
D = Severe	4 = Most of the time
C = Moderate	3 = Some of the time
B = Slight	2 = Hardly at all
A = No symptom	1 = Not at all

* Adpated from Erskine and Schonell, 1979.

Table 4-2

DAILY SYMPTOM QUESTIONNAIRE*

		Days: 1	2	3	4	5	6	7
Had an attack?	Yes or No							
Severity of attack	Severity scale							
Duration of attack	Frequency scale							
Wheeze?	Yes or No							
Severity of wheeze	Severity scale							
Duration of wheeze	Frequency scale							
No. of times woken during the night								
No. of times used inhaler								
Interfered with normal activities	Frequency scale							
Did you have to call the doctor?	Yes No							

SCALES

Severity	*Frequency*
E = Very severe	5 = All of the time
D = Severe	4 = Most of the time
C = Moderate	3 = Some of the time
B = Slight	2 = Hardly at all

* Adapted from Erskine and Schonell, 1979.

patients (20 to 30 minutes, two times per day for three months). Schaeffer and Freytag-Klinger (1975) successfully used autogenic training to treat asthma patients.

Sirota and Mahoney (1974) combined the use of cue-controlled relaxation with gradual reduction in bronchometer use to successfully treat one asthmatic patient. They describe the use of the procedure as follows:

> She was given a portable timer to carry at all times. For the first 5 days she was to set the timer for semi-random intervals averaging 30 minutes in length. When the timer buzzed, the client was briefly to inventory her muscles for tension, note her anxiety level, and relax away any incipient tension. . . . The timer interval was subsequently lengthened to 1 hour. An additional treatment strategy (begun on day 9) involved brief postponement of bronchometer use. Any time Mrs. W. experienced breathing difficulty and wanted to use her inhalant, she was to set the timer for 3-4 min, practice an abbreviated (four muscle group) relaxation, and to then employ the bronchometer only if necessary. . . . A total of nine therapy sessions were given. [pp. 65-66]

Systematic desensitization has been the most frequently used treatment technique and has generally been found to be superior to the use of relaxation alone. Systematic desensitization has generally been done to internal stimuli, such as symptoms and thoughts during an attack (e.g., fighting for breath) or external stimuli, such as the circumstances and precipitants of an attack (e.g., a very hot day in a closed room), or both. Moore (1965) provides the following excellent examples of the first type of hierarchy:

HIERARCHY

This is based on an asthmatic attack and is given to all patients in the same form.

1. **Very slight wheeze**
2. **Just a bit more wheezy**
3. **Wheezy, uncomfortable lying down**
4. **Very wheezy and have to sit up**
5. **Quite wheezy even sitting up in bed**
6. **Very wheezy even sitting up**
7. **Difficult to get the breath**
8. **Feel you cannot breathe**
9. **Fighting for breath**
10. **Cannot go on fighting, feel as if you are going to die**

[p. 271]

Yorkston, McHugh, Brady, Serber, and Sergeant (1974) describe a systematic desensitization program that incorporates both the symptoms of an attack and individual precipitants and thoughts of an attack.

Symptoms of Asthma or Tension

(i) Standard description. This was given sentence by sentence to every patient.

Breathlessness. **"Everyone has felt a little breathless at some time in his life. Everyone knows what it is like to feel breathless, for example, when he hurries. Everyone knows what it is like to feel breathless. Everyone has felt breathless. Sometimes I feel breathless. Like everyone else, I expect that you sometimes feel breathless. Sometimes you feel breathless." A similar sequence was followed for the phrases "very breathless," "difficulty catching your breath," "difficulty in breathing out," "your breath is prolonged," and "you feel you can't get your next breath out," leading to "sometines you have difficulty breathig out and your breath is prolonged" . . .**

Wheezing. **"Sometimes you wheeze (feel breathless and wheeze; feel very breathless and wheeze loudly)."**

Tightness. **. . . "We use our chests to breathe. Sometimes we are aware of our breathing (I am; you are). Sometimes you are aware of your chest while you are breathing. Sometimes your chest feels a little uncomfortable (a little tight; tight; very tight). Sometimes you feel breathless, feel tight in the chest, and wheeze."**

Palpitations. **"Everyone knows what it is like to feel his heart beating. Sometimes when we hurry we feel our hearts beating (I; you). Sometimes when you feel breathless you feel your heart beating. Sometimes you feel very tight in the chest, feel you can't get your next breath out, and feel your heart beating."**

Tension. . . . "When something unusual happens, our natural reaction is to become alert. If something unusual happens in our bodies, we naturally become alert and notice what is happening. If we get breathless, we naturally notice what is happening. If we get breathless, we naturally notice it. When you get breathless (tight in the chest; wheeze), you notice it. If we notice something going wrong, we naturally become alert and brace ourselves to deal with the situation. If we notice something inside us changing, we often react naturally by becoming alert and bracing ourselves. When we become alert and brace ourselves, we often become tense. Everyone knows what it is like to feel tense (I; you). Sometimes when you get breathless and wheeze and feel tight in the chest, you feel tense and anxious."

Other specific symptoms. Autonomic or other specific symptoms were treated in a similar way: with a general proposition, followed by statements that I have it, that you probably have it, that you do have it, and that you have it with other symptoms. Asthma. The word "asthma" was often provocative and so it was avoided until this stage when it was at first embedded in neutral or positive statements. "It is one of the facts of life that there is a disorder called asthma. A great deal of work is being undertaken to help people with asthma. It is a fact that you have asthma."

The word "asthma" was then linked with its symptoms: "Sometimes you feel breathless when you get asthma (tight in the chest; anxious; tense). Sometimes you feel very breathless, tight in the chest, anxious and tense when you have asthma."

(ii) Personal description. The individual's description of his attack of asthma was given phrase by phrase, starting with the prodromal symptoms, for example, "An early sign of asthma is feeling a little tight in the chest." When the patient had adapted to each fragment of history, the components of the attack were successively combined until he could listen quite calmly to a full description of it.

Thoughts during an attack

Similarly, the patient was desensitized to his disturbing thoughts one by one, from the least to the most distressing. These were then combined with the description of the asthmatic attack until the patient could think calmly about the attack and his worst thoughts in it, for example, "You sometimes wonder if you are going to die."

Circumstances of the attack

The circumstances in which asthmatic attacks occurred were grouped by theme and ranked from the least to the most disturbing. Beginning with the least provocative item, the patient was desensitized to each in turn. Later, descriptions of the circumstances, the attacks, and the thoughts and feelings during the attacks were given in combination.

(5) Practical desensitization

When the patient had been desensitized verbally, he could think calmly about his asthma, its circumstances, and the thoughts and feelings it evoked. He was then encouraged to relax himself in everyday life before gradually facing any circumstances which he had previously avoided. [pp. 372-373]

Yorkston et al. (1974) found that the greatest improvements with their patients occurred between sessions. Therefore, it may be more effective to space out the systematic desensitization sessions. Yorkston, Eckert, McHugh, Philander, and Blumenthal (1979) also successfully used the following type of practical desensitization with asthmatic patients:

> **[The practical desensitization] was aimed at desensitizing the patients to expiratory effort by having them gradually accustom themselves to making graduated expiratory efforts without provoking tension. This was done by having each patient expire against increasing resistance through a tube into a blow-bottle containing colored water. The out-flow tube of this blow-bottle was 0.5 cm in internal diameter and was one meter high. Each patient was encouraged to progress at his or her own rate to blow and sustain the column of colored water to as high a level as possible during the time available. [p. 326]**

No difference was found between practical and verbal desensitization. However, only patients taking steroids generally benefited from the desensitization. If the results of the assessment revealed other anxiety arousing themes or phobias, it may be useful to desensitize patients to these themes (e.g., anger, fear of failure, or fear of being alone).

Other behavioral techniques have been attempted on a very limited basis. MacDonald and Oden (1977) successfully used a reinforcement program of rewarding two patients daily for not having attacks. Assertive training has been used by Walton (1960) to treat an asthma patient whose attacks were related to anxiety in his relationships with other people.

Biofeedback has also been occasionally used with asthma patients. Lerro, Hurnyak, and Patterson (1980) used thermal biofeedback to successfully treat one patient. Vachon and Rich (1976) and Steptoe, Phillips, and Harling (1981) successfully used feedback of respiratory resistance with some asthma patients.

For More Information

Erskine-Milliss, J., & Schonell, M. (1981). Relaxation therapy in asthma: A critical review. *Psychosomatic Medicine, 43*, 365-372.

This article reviews the treatments of relaxation therapy, systematic desensitization, and biofeedback with both adult and child asthma patients. It contains a good introduction explaining both the psychological and physiological factors involved in asthma. The article can be obtained from Professor M. Schonell, The St. George Hospital, Kogarah, NSW, 2217, Australia.

Knapp, T., & Wells, L. (1978). Behavior therapy for asthma: A review. *Behavior Research and Therapy, 16*, 103-115.

This article provides an excellent review of both the physiological and self-report assessment techniques. All of the different behavioral treatment techniques are reviewed for both adult and child patients. The article can be obtained from Terry J. Knapp, Department of Psychology, University of Nevada, Las Vegas, NV 89154.

Yorkston, V., McHugh, R., Brady, R., Serber, M., & Sergeant, H. (1974). Verbal desensitisation in bronchial asthma. *Journal of Psychosomatic Research, 18*, 371-376.

This study provides a detailed description of the desensitization procedure that was successfully used to treat six asthma patients. The article can be obtained from N.J. Yorkston, Friern Hospital, London N.11, England or from H.G.S.

Sergeant, University of Minnesota, Minneapolis, MN.

References

Erskine, J., & Schonell, M. (1979). Relaxation therapy in bronchial asthma. *Journal of Psychosomatic Research, 23*, 131-139.

Knapp, T., & Wells, L. (1978). Behavior therapy for asthma: A review. *Behavioral Research and Therapy, 16*, 103-115.

Lerro, F., Hurnyak, M., & Patterson, C. (1980). Successful use of thermal biofeedback in severe adult asthma. *American Journal of Psychiatry, 137*, 735-736.

MacDonald, W., & Oden, C. (1977). Role clarification and sanction in two cases of bronchial asthma. *The Journal of Asthma Research, 14*, 189-197.

Mathison, D. (1976). In H.F. Conn (Ed.), *Current Therapy* (pp. 574-579). Philadelphia: Saunders.

Moore, N. (1965). Behaviour therapy in bronchial asthma: A controlled study. *Journal of Psychosomatic Research, 9*, 257-276.

Phillip, R., Wilde, G., & Day, J. (1972). Suggestion and relaxation in asthmatics. *Journal of Psychosomatic Research, 16*, 193-204.

Schaeffer, G., & Freytag-Klinger, H. (1975). Objectifying the effect of autogenic training on disordered ventilation in bronchial asthma. *Psychiatry, Neurology, Medicine, Psychology* (Leipz), *27*, 400-408.

Sirota, A., & Mahoney, M. (1974). Relaxing on cue: The self regulation of asthma. *Journal of Behavior Therapy and Experimental Psychiatry, 5*, 65-66.

Steptoe, A., Phillips, J., & Harling, J. (1981). Biofeedback and instructions in the modification of total respiratory resistance: An experimental study of asthmatic and non-asthmatic volunteers. *Journal of Psychosomatic Research, 25*, 541-551.

Vachon, L., & Rich, E. (1976). Visceral learning in asthma. *Psychosomatic Medicine, 38*, 122-130.

Walton, D. (1960). The application of learning theory to the treatment of a case of bronchial asthma. In H.J. Eysenck (Ed.), *Behavior Therapy* (pp. 188-189). New York: Pergamon Press.

Wilson, A., Honsberger, R., Chiu, J., & Novey, H. (1975). Transcendental meditation and asthma. *Respiration, 32*, 75-80.

Yorkston, N., Eckert, E., McHugh, R., Philander, D., & Blumenthal, M. (1979). Bronchial asthma: Improved lung function after behavior modification. *Psychosomatics, 20*, 325-331.

Yorkston, N., McHugh, R., Brady, R., Serber, M., & Sergeant, H. (1974). Verbal desensitization in bronchial asthma. *Journal of Psychosomatic Research, 18*, 371-376.

5 Blepharospasm

Assessment Strategies

Blepharospasm is a severe eye blink tic. The disorder has been associated with many organic causes, including Parkinson's disease and tardive dyskinesia. Therefore, a thorough medical evaluation is suggested before implementing any behavioral treatment. A behavioral assessment should involve a time-sampled frequency count of the patient by an observer. Additionally, an ABC behavioral diary, including ratings and severity of the tic, will aid in selecting the treatment strategy. A general measure of anxiety (e.g., State-Trait Anxiety Inventory) may also be useful.

Treatment Strategies

The reported behavioral treatment of blepharospasm is limited to a few case studies. Most of the case studies tend to combine treatment approaches. For those patients who demonstrate a generally high level of anxiety, relaxation training may have some impact on the tic. Patients should be instructed not to force open their eyelids during a spasm. They should try to relax and let the eyelids open spontaneously. If increased blepharospasm is related to anxiety-provoking situations, as determined by the behavioral diary, systematic desensitization should be included in the treatment package.

Beck and Fedoravicius (1977) combined relaxation training, assertiveness training, and spouse reinforcement with a procedure designed to increase the patient's eye blink control. They describe the eye blink control procedure as follows:

> **The procedure consisted of having the patient stare at selected objects in the office without blinking while the therapist counted out 3 sec. Following the count of three the patient was instructed to blink once. This procedure was practiced during the first and last 10 min of each session. During the fourth and subsequent treatment sessions the patient assumed the counting responsibilities while staring at objects in the room. Additionally, during the fourth session he was instructed to count to five before blinking and to subvocalize the counting. [p. 278]**

For some patients it is necessary to develop reinforcing situations where their eyes can remain open. Additionally, some patients may need to have their eyelid movements gradually retrained. Sharpe (1974) describes the general retraining as follows:

> **The eyelid movements were gradually retrained through exercises from gross movements to progressively more refined control. Thus, initially he squeezed his eyes shut and then relaxed them; then he imagined opening his eyes; then he opened and closed his eyes; then he blinked his eyes for longer and longer periods; then he held them one "hooded" or half open; then he winked them independently; then he moved them normally. [pp. 603-604]**

Massed practice is another technique used in most treatment packages. Massed practice for blepharospasm involves having the patient deliberately blink while looking in the mirror. Massed practice sessions from two to six minutes have been used. It may be appropriate to start with a two-minute session alternating with a one- or two-minute rest period, and by the second or third session to have five or six minutes of massed practice alternating with one minute of rest. A total of 30 minutes of massed practice during a session should be sufficient. Additionally, the patient should practice the massed practice at home, at least twice daily.

It is important to tell the patient to increase the effort of the eye blink response on each succeeding trial during the sessions. If massed practice is successful, a sharp improvement in the frequency of the tic may be seen in the first few days of treatment.

For More Information

Frederick, C. (1971). Treatment of a tic by systematic desensitization and massed response evocation. *Journal of Behavior Therapy and Experimental Psychiatry, 2*, 281-283.

This case study contains a good description of the massed practice procedure and its combined clinical use with systematic desensitization. The article can be obtained from Calvin J. Frederick, Center for Studies of Suicide Prevention, Department of Health, Education and Welfare, 5600 Fishers Lane, Rockville, MD 20852.

Sharpe, R. (1974). Behaviour therapy in a case of blepharospasm. *British Journal of Psychiatry, 124*, 603-604.

This case study combines relaxation therapy, reinforcement, and eyelid movement retraining in the treatment of blepharospasm. The article can be obtained from Robert Sharpe, Ph.D., Center Director, Center for Behavioral Psychotherapy, 38 Weymouth St., London, W1N3LR, England.

References

Beck, S., & Fedoravicius, A. (1977). Self-control treatment of an eye blink tic. *Behavior Therapy, 8*, 275-277.

Sharpe, R. (1974). Behaviour therapy in a case of blepharospasm. *British Journal of Psychiatry, 124*, 603-604.

6 Bulimia

Assessment Strategies

Bulimia is an eating disorder characterized by binge eating often followed by self-induced vomiting or laxative use. A thorough medical assessment should precede the behavioral assessment. A one- or two-week baseline period is suggested prior to selecting an intervention strategy.

The most common behavioral assessment involves a food diary that consists of a record of all episodes of bingeing, vomiting, and laxative use. A typical behavioral analysis diary is shown.

Additionally, some clinicians have monitored daily intake, the patient's daily weight, exercise activity, and the number of calories vomited daily (measured as the sum of all calories consumed 1 1/2 hours prior to vomiting).

An alternative behavioral measure is a test meal. Leiterberg, Gross, Peterson, and Rosen (1984) describe the procedure as follows:

> **Subjects were instructed to eat these test meals by themselves and to try to eat as much as they could keep down knowing in advance that they were not supposed to vomit for 2 1/2 hours afterwards. They were also instructed to eat what they normally would prior to the time of these test meals but not to vomit for 1 1/2 hours beforehand.**
>
> **One food from each of the three targeted food groups (large meal, sweets/snack food, pasta) was chosen as a standard stimulus for each subject. For example, for subject 1, the large test meal consisted of a 4 oz.hamburger, 1/2 cup cooked vegetables, 1 pint tossed salad, 1 baked potato, and 2 slices of bread; sweets consisted of 3 candy bars; and pasta consisted of 1 quart of spaghetti with tomato sauce. [p. 9]**

Checklists and rating scales can also be used to assess bulimia. The Eating Attitudes Test is a 40-item questionnaire which measures the following factors: food preoccupation, body-image for thinness, vomiting and laxative abuse, dieting, slow eating, clandestine eating, and perceived pressure to gain weight (Garner & Garfinkel, 1979).

The Eating Habits Checklist (Gormally, Black, Daston & Rardin, 1982) is a 16-item scale that assesses the behavioral manifestations of a binge and the thoughts that precipitate and follow a binge.

Hawkins and Clement (1980) have developed a 19-item scale that measures binge eating. Table 6-1 lists typical items from the scale.

Smith and Thelen (1984) developed a 32-item questionnaire, The Bulimia Test (Bulit), to

> **(a) . . . distinguish between individuals who exhibit the bulimia syndrome and individuals with no eating problems, (b) distinguish between bulimic individuals and those with other eating disorders, (c) distinguish between subgroups of bulimics based on particular criteria (e.g., severity of vomiting, purging, and fasting behaviors), and (d) provide these distinctions for individuals who have never soughts treatment as well as for those who have. [p. 864]**

Date Time	What was happening before the binge?	Binge foods eaten and quantity	Where eaten	Other people present	Consequences-feelings and thoughts after binging	Amount of time after binge to vomit	Consequences-feelings and thoughts after vomiting

Figure 6-1

Behavioral Analysis for Bulimia

Table 6-1

NINE ITEMS FROM THE BINGE SCALE QUESTIONNAIRE

1. ***How often do you binge eat?***
a. seldom b. once or twice month c. once a week d. almost every day.

Scores: a (0); b (1); c (2); d (3).

2. ***What is the average length of a binge eating episode?***
a. less than 15 minutes b. 15 minutes to one hour
c. one hour to four hours d. more than four hours.

Scores: a (0); b (1); c (2); d (3).

3. ***Which of the following statements best applies to your binge eating?***
a. I eat until I have had enough to satisfy me. b. I eat until my stomach feels full.
c. I eat until my stomach is painfully full. d. I eat until I can't eat anymore.

Scores: a (0); b (1); c (2); d (3).

4. ***Do you ever vomit after a binge?***
a. never b. sometimes c. usually d. always.

Scores: a (0); b (1); c (2); d (3).

5. ***Which of the following best applies to your eating behavior when binge eating?***
a. I eat more slowly than usual. b. I eat about the same as I usually do.
c. I eat very rapidly.

Scores: a (0); b (0); c (1).

6. ***How much are you concerned about your binge eating?***
a. not bothered at all. b. bothers me a little c. moderately concerned
d. a major concern.

Scores: a (0); b (1); c (2); d (3).

7. ***Which best describes your feelings during a binge?***
a. I feel that I could control the eating if I chose.
b. I feel that I have at least some control. c. I feel completely out of control.

Scores: a (0); b (1); c (2).

8. ***Which of the following describes your feelings after a binge?***
a. I feel fairly neutral, not too concerned. b. I am moderately upset.
c. I hate myself.

Scores: a (0); b (1); c (2).

9. ***Which most accurately describes your feelings after a binge?***
a. not depressed at all b. mildly depressed c. moderately depressed
d. very depressed.

Scores: a (0); b (1); c (2); d (3).

[Hawkins & Clement, 1980; p. 221]

The Eating Disorders Inventory is a 64-item self-report measure. This inventory consists of thoughts often associated with anorexia nervosa and bulimia (Garner, Olmstead, & Polivy, 1983).

The Bulimia Cognitive Distortions Scale is a 25-item inventory that measures irrational beliefs and cognitive distortions associated with bulimia (Schulman, Kider, Powers, Prange, & Gleghorn, 1986).

Many bulimic patients often experience depression. Therefore, it may be useful to include a short measure of depression (e.g. Beck Depression Inventory) during the assessment.

Treatment Strategies

Continuation of the food diaries during treatment will aid in monitoring treatment progress. Educating the patient on the dangers of vomiting and laxative abuse is an important early step in treatment. Giles, Young, and Young (1984) give the patient the following information:

> 1. **Dieting causes metabolic rate to diminish.**
> 2. **The carbohydrate molecule is infused with an abundance of oxygen atoms; consequently, the body uses this oxygen to metabolize its food (versus storing carbohydrates as fat).**
> 3. **Bingeing, even when followed by vomiting, exposes the binger to hundreds of calories because simple carbohydrates are absorbed into the blood stream in as little as 10-15 minutes.**
> 4. **Only 66% of the carbohydrate is assimilated by the body (versus 75% to 80% for fats and protein). The rest is excreted.**
> 5. **Strict abstinence from a particular food group may induce craving for that group.**
> 6. **Most moderately active young women metabolize 1,700- 2,200 calories per day. Therefore, doughnuts, candy bars, ice cream, and so on are not fattening as long as this calorie range is maintained.**
> 7. **It usually requires 3,500 extra calories for one pound of body weight to occur.**
> 8. **Rapid weight loss usually entails 50% fluid loss (rapidly regained), 25% muscle tissue (causing less muscle tone and less capacity to metabolize calories), and only 25% fat. It was further explained that, for most people, only one to two pounds of fat can be lost per week.**
> 9. **The anxiety and urge to vomit after feeling full, eating too much, eating non-diet foods, and so on,declines significantly, usually within an hour, even if no vomiting occurs.**
> 10. **Fear of food greatly diminishes when one stays within a normal caloric range (versus dieting) long enough to see that a reasonable weight is maintained. [pp. 396-397]**

The most widely used behavioral treatments for bulimia are exposure and response prevention, and stimulus control. In the exposure and response prevention treatment, the patient can be told that binge eating is being maintained by the vomiting. Learning to control the vomiting will enable the patient to control the binge eating. Leitenberg et al. (1984) describe the exposure and response prevention procedure as follows:

> Each treatment session had two basic parts: (a) exposure to the feared stimulus, i.e., eating particular foods or particular amounts of food; (b) prevention of the habitual escape response, i.e., vomiting. During each treatment session subjects were instructed to eat an amount of food which caused a strong urge to vomit, past the point where vomiting would ordinarily occur. The specific food items within a group varied across subjects, the choices depending on what they found most anxiety provoking. The amount of food provided within each food group, however, was constant across subjects, e.g., when candy bars were used, 3 were provided each time; pasta could be either 1 quart of spaghetti or 3 slices of pizza from the same take-out restaurant; pastry could be 3 doughnuts or 3 brownies, etc. These amounts could be considered within or slightly above the range most people could eat comfortably. Extremely large amounts were intentionally avoided and unnecessary, because in the absence of vomiting, even very small quantities of these foods (e.g., two bites of a brownie) could provoke intense anxiety. . . . The subjects were told that they would not be allowed to vomit immediately after eating, and that the therapist would stay with them until the urge to vomit was under control. They were also told that treatment would be most beneficial if they did not vomit within 2 1/2 hours after the end of any treatment session, and that it was best to stay with the therapist until they felt they could safely leave without vomiting afterwards.
>
> In each therapy session, the therapist tried to direct the subject's attention to whatever anxiety-provoking thoughts and feelings were induced while eating. These usually centered around negative body image, sensations of feeling full, gross, fat, wanting to vomit, fears of weight gain and binge-eating in public, and relationship issues with spouses, parents, friends, and co-workers, including themes of anger, loss, and rejection.
>
> During sessions when bulimia nervosa patients were repeatedly exposed to eating without vomiting, the therapist tried to help the patient make several discoveries:
>
> 1. In the absence of planned vomiting they do not have an uncontrollable craving to consume huge amounts of food; instead they have an obsessive craving to be slim, to eat as little as possible, to not gain weight;
> 2. Physical sensations of immediate weight gain and feelings of gross changes in bodily appearance (particularly stomach, thighs, and buttocks) following consumption of normal or even less than normal amounts of food are distorted, and these feelings are capable of being relieved without recourse to vomiting;
> 3. They are able to eat certain foods without "having to" vomit afterwards;
> 4. The anxiety they experience after eating forbidden foods is not as overwhelming as they first thought it would be and is capable of diminishing to tolerable levels even if they do not vomit;
> 5. Their desire to maintain a strict diet and their criteria of "bad" foods, "having eaten too much," "having blown it" are distorted and serve to trigger the impulse to eat even more and to vomit afterwards;
> 6. The obsessive desire to achieve a "perfect" slim body usually stems from a complex mix of disturbed family relationships, low self-esteem, and associated fears of rejection and abandonment, a variety of guilt feelings, and cultural values and stereotyped beliefs about appropriate feminine appearance and behavior. Therapy sessions were conducted at a set time of day for each subject, either at noon or 6 p.m. The length of each treatment session varied, depending on how long it took for a subject's urge to vomit to decline to negligible levels. [pp. 6-7]

During exposure and response prevention patients should frequently rate their anxiety, on a SUDS scale, and rate the urge to vomit on a 0-to-100 scale. Patients can be asked to bring different foods to the session, beginning with the least difficult and progressing to the most difficult. The type and amount of food can be negotiated with the therapist. Sessions can also be conducted in the environment (e.g., cafeteria) with therapist modeling. Between sessions the patient can be instructed to practice the exposure and response prevention daily. It is also possible to train significant others to supervise the home practice. With this type of treatment it is common for anxiety and the urge to vomit to increase during the session before eventually declining. However, anxiety and the urge to vomit generally decrease across sessions.

Cinciripini, Kornblith, Turner, and Hersen (1983) combined exposure to binge foods with verbal flooding of the bulimic act in treating a bulimic patient. They also required the patient to purchase food items or to enter stores where binge items were available.

Stimulus control techniques have also been frequently used with bulimic patients. Kirkley, Schneider, Agras, and Bachman (1985) describe a treatment package consisting of several stimulus control techniques as follows:

> **(a) . . . increase eating regularity (i.e., move closer to three to five meals per day); (b) delay vomiting by gradually increasing the time between bingeing and vomiting and using incompatible behaviors to achieve this; (c) increase the variety of foods eaten to include foods from all the major food groups, particularly eating previously feared and avoided foods; (d) decrease eating rate; (e) eat only when sitting at a table and using utensils; (f) alter their vomiting ritual in some way; (g) eat "forbidden foods" in nonbinge settings; and (h) use relaxation tapes. [p. 45]**

Stimulus control can also be used to physically restrict thepatient from access to certain situations (e.g., the kitchen), or to limit foods and situations related to vomiting. Stimulus narrowing (i.e., eating only during prescribed times) alone has not been found to be effective (Mizes & Lohr, 1983).

Cognitive restructuring techniques have been found to be helpful in combination with the exposure and response prevention techniques (Wilson, Rossiter, Klefield, & Lindholm, 1986).

Cognitive restructuring has also been successfully combined with stimulus control techniques (Grine, 1982; Schneider & Agras, 1983). The techniques have generally focused on the patient's irrational concerns about weight, body image, and rigid rules about eating. Cognitive restructuring and stimulus-control procedures used together have also been successfully used in group treatment of bulimics. Schneider and Agras (1985) describe a three-phase, 16-session group procedure as follows:

> **Phase I: Sessions 1-5. Phase I aimed at establishing group cohesion and disclosure of the eating and vomiting rituals, while at the same time exploring the behavioural and cognitive functions served by these behaviours. Emphasis was placed on becoming aware of current behaviours. Participants were cautioned against trying to make rapid rather than small, gradual changes. The goals of Phase I were accomplished through self-monitoring of eating and vomiting behaviours as well as the events, cognitions, and affective states that preceded or followed them. Affective expression was encouraged, and this facilitated the understanding of faulty beliefs**

> **related to bulimic behaviours. Attention was also given to the importance of eating regular, balanced meals. This was done through discussion of nutrition and examination of each patient's definition of diets, binges, and regular eating patterns. Each week, suggestions were developed toward making changes in these areas.**
>
> **Phase II: Sessions 5-10. Phase II of the treatment dealt with exploration of behaviours, cognitions, and affects associated with out-of-control eating. The treatment became more individualised in terms of interpersonal problem-solving, related to deficient assertive skills. Coping strategies were explored that would help deal with boredom resulting from the unstructured time necessary in developing greater self-control. More attention was focused on actual vomiting behaviours and on the rituals surrounding them. Binge guidelines were suggested that would enhance self-control, including the delay of impulses to binge by increments of five, then ten minutes, then examining cognitive and affective states during the delay period; extending the time between eating binge foods; limiting the length of binges; and changing eating patterns—sitting at the kitchen table rather than eating from an open refrigerator, food boxes, or counter tops, or leaving the kitchen and/or house immediately after eating. Watching television and eating were eliminated from the binge cycle, to allow patients to concentrate on bodily hunger signals. A three-part relaxation program . . . was included to reduce stress and anxiety and enhance self-control. Initial practice took place in the group, and patients were then given three relaxation tapes (one every two weeks) for daily home practice. These exercises also provided an additional coping strategy for handling urges to binge.**
>
> **Phase III: Sessions 11-16. During this third phase, patients were encouraged to take more responsibility for their behaviour and to begin setting individual weekly goals around eating behaviour and social activities. Attention was directed toward the development of more assertive behaviours, and this was accomplished by supportive challenges to distorted cognitions. The introduction of previously forbidden foods into diets was discussed and considered. Unrealistic expectations regarding sudden weight gain when vomiting ceased was dealt with through the reported successful experiences of other group members. [pp. 67-68]**

If the assessment reveals that the major antecedent for bulimic behavior is weight loss, it may be necessary to teach the patient appropriate weight loss strategies. Relaxation or stress management techniques may be necessary if anxiety is an antecedent of bulimic behaviors. Similarly, treatment for depression may be indicated if depressive feelings precede bingeing. Assertiveness training is indicated if the assessment reveals that the patient's inability to deal with other people leads to bingeing.

Thought stopping has not been found to be helpful in eliminating bulimic behaviors (Cinciripini et al., 1983).

For More Information

Johnson, C., Connors, M., & Tobin, D. (1987). Symptom management of bulimia. *Journal of Consulting and Clinical Psychology, 55*, 668-676.

This article describes a treatment program for bulimia that includes education, self-monitoring, stimulus control, and cognitive restructuring. Included is a discussion of techniques that can be used to regulate mood. The article can be obtained from Craig Johnson, Eating Disorders Program, Northwestern Memorial Hospital, 320 East Huron, Second Floor, Chicago, IL 60611.

Orleans, C., & Barnett, L. (1980, November). *Bulimarexia guidelines for behavioral assessment and treatment*. Paper presented at the meeting of the Association for Advancement of Behavior Therapy, New York, N.Y.

This paper defines the problem and includes some data on prevalence and patient characteristics. Additionally, a theoretical analysis of the problem is discussed. Specific behavior assessment guidelines and treatment strategies are elucidated. The paper can be obtained from C. Tracy Orleans, Medical Psychology, Box 3837, Duke University Medical Center, Durham, NC 27710.

Schlesler-Stropp, B. (1984). Bulimia: A review of the literature. *Psychological Bulletin, 95*, 247-257.

This article initially reviews the diagnosis, incidence and demographic variables of bulimia. The psychopathology and physiological factors are reviewed. Behavioral and non-behavioral treatments are also reviewed. The article can be obtained from Barbara Schlesler-Stroop, University of Southern Mississippi, SS Box 5012, Hattlesburg, Miss. 39406.

Wilson, G. (1986). Cognitive-behavioral and pharmacological therapies for bulimia. In K. Brownell & J. Foreyt (Eds.) *Handbook of Eating Disorders* (pp. 450-475). New York: Basic Books.

This chapter reviews the uncontrolled clinical reports, controlled outcome studies, and single-case experimental studies of the cognitive-behavioral treatment of bulimia. Included are practical techniques and a section on pharmacological treatments. The book can be obtained from Basic Books, 10 E. 53rd Street, New York, NY 10022.

References

Cinciripini, P., Kornblith, S., Turner, S., & Hersen, M. (1983). A behavioral program for the management of anorexia and bulimia. *The Journal of Nervous and Mental Disease, 171*, 186-189.

Garner, D., & Garfinkel, P. (1979). The Eating Attitudes Test: An index of the symptoms of anorexia nervosa. *Psychosomatic Medicine, 9* 273-279.

Garner, D., Olmstead, M., & Polivy, J. (1983). Development and validation of a multidimensional eating disorder inventory for anorexia nervosa and bulimia. *International Journal of Eating Disorders, 2*, 15-35.

Giles, T., Young, R., & Young, D. (1985). Behavioral treatment of severe bulimia. *Behavior Therapy, 16*, 393-405.

Gormally, J., Black, S., Daston, S., & Rardin, D. (1982). The assessment of binge eating severity among obese persons. *Addictive Behaviors, 7*, 47-55.

Grinc, G. (1982). A cognitive-behavioral model for the treatment of chronic vomiting. *Journal of Behavioral Medicine, 5*, 135-141.

Hawkins, R., & Clement, P. (1980). Development in construct validation of a self-report measure of binge eating tendencies. *Addictive Behaviors, 5*, 219-226.

Kirkley, B., Schneider, J., Agras, W., & Bachman, J. (1985). Comparison of two group treatments for bulimia. *Journal of Consulting and Clinical Psychology, 53*, 43-48.

Leitenberg, H., Gross, J., Peterson, J., & Rosen, J. (1984). Analysis of an anxiety model in the process of change during exposure plus response prevention treatment of bulimia nervosa. *Behavior Therapy, 15*, 3-20.

Mizes, J., & Lohr, J. (1983). The treatment of bulimia (binge-eating and self-induced vomiting): A quasi-experimental investigation of the effects of stimulus narrowing, self-reinforcement and self-control relaxation. *International Journal of Eating Disorders, 2*, 59-65.

Schneider, J., & Agras, W. (1985). A cognitive behavioural group treatment of bulimia. *British Journal of Psychiatry, 146*, 66-69.

Schulman, R., Kinder, B., Powers, M., Prange, M., & Gleghorn, A. The development of a scale to measure cognitive distortions in bulimia. *Journal of Personality Assessment, 50*, 630-639.

Smith, M., & Thelen, M. (1984). Development and validation of a test for bulimia. *Journal of Consulting and Clinical Psychology, 52*, 863-872.

Wilson, G., Rossiter, E., Kleifield, E., & Lindholm, L. (1986). Cognitive-behavioral treatment of bulimia nervosa: A controlled evaluation. *Behavior Research and Therapy, 24*, 277-288.

See Also

Chapter 1: Anorexia Nervosa

7 Bruxism

Assessment Strategies

Bruxism is a non-functional clenching or grinding of the teeth, or both, that can occur when the person is awake or asleep. Some of the symptoms indicative of clenching are sore, fatigued jaw muscles while chewing, pain in the jaw muscles, the ear, or the temporomandibular joint. Night-time bruxism usually can be detected by another person who reports grinding noises. Often the nighttime bruxer will awaken with tooth pain or stiff jaw muscles, or both. The condition is generally diagnosed by dentists.

The easiest monitoring consists of having the patient record, on a wrist counter, tally sheet, or index card the number of grinding incidents per day. A one- to two-week baseline should be sufficient. For nighttime bruxism, the patient should audiotape a sample of sleep each night to determine frequency. More accurate assessment and monitoring devices are available (e.g., EMG biofeedback). However, these devices may be expensive and may interfere with the patient's normal pattern of sleep or activity.

Treatment Strategies

The first attempt at treatment should involve self-monitoring. To make self-monitoring as accurate as possible, the patient should describe the response in detail to the therapist and then demonstrate the response. Additionally, the patient should learn to detect the occurrence of the earliest sign of the response (e.g., jaw movement). This self-monitoring may be all that is needed to stop the habit for some patients. Jenkins and Peterson (1978) have increased the effectiveness of the self-monitoring by adding the adversive stimulus of a squirt of lemon juice contingent on tooth grinding. If two weeks of self-monitoring is not effective in reducing bruxism, other techniques may be added.

Massed practice can be easily added to the self-monitoring program. The patient should be instructed to clench his or her teeth together tightly and then to relax the jaws. What may be critical to the success of this technique is the amount of time the patient practices the response. Although many patients have been successful with short time periods (i.e., five seconds of clenching followed by five seconds of relaxation, repeated five times), it appears that a fatigue level should be established for each patient individually. Some patients may need one minute or more of continued clenching. Each of the blocks of trials should be repeated approximately six times per day. If the technique is successful, a change in the grinding habit should take place in about ten days to two weeks. It is important to have the patient continue monitoring progress during this time. Some possible problems with massed practice include the occurrence of pain if the practice is used for extended periods of time. In addition, some patients may view the technique as adversive and will not comply. Finally, the technique is not indicated for patients who have facial pain.

Habit reversal has also been used successfully in treating bruxism (Rosenbaum & Aylon, 1981). The treatment begins with the response description and early warning procedures that were previously mentioned in regard to self-monitoring. By keeping track of the details of the situations that elicit the behavior in a behavioral diary, the patient is made aware of their occurrence. The negative aspects of the behavior are discussed with the therapist and then a competing response procedure is initiated. An isometric type exercise (e.g., opening the mouth) that is incompatible with the bruxism behavior is used. The exercise should be practiced for about one minute and should be socially inconspicuous. It should be practiced after any urge, any noticeable antecedent, or after the occurrence of the behavior.

A covert rehearsal of a typical situation where the patient may grind his or her teeth should be practiced in the office, several times, with the therapist. This treatment may be successful after a one-hour therapy session. Stress management may be another successful approach. Relaxation training alone has generally not been successful. However, if it is determined that the patient is anxious, a stress reduction program which includes relaxation training may be appropriate. The inclusion of cognitive techniques that focus on thoughts of the patient during times of stress can also be included. A covert rehearsal technique may be useful. Have the patient imagine a stressful situation and repeat appropriate statements (e.g., "I can handle this" or "Just relax") out loud. The patient should then monitor his or her thoughts during real life situations. Biofeedback should also be considered for this problem and may be especially helpful for the patient who experiences the problem only at night (e.g., Cassisi & McGlynn, 1988). The general procedure involves an audible tone that is sounded if the patient clenches or grinds his or her teeth during the night. Small portable EMG devices are available for this type of biofeedback treatment.

For More Information

Bailey, J.O., & Rugh, J.D. (1979). Behavior management of functional oral disorders. In P. Bryant, E.N. Gale, & J.D. Rugh (Eds.), *Oral motor behavior: Impact on oral conditions and dental treatment* (NIH Pub. No. 79-1845). Washington: U.S. Government Printing Office.

This article reviews the biofeedback and behavioral treatment approaches to bruxism. It can be obtained from the U.S. Government Printing Office, Washington, D.C.

Glaros, A.G., & Ral, S.M. (1977). Bruxism: A critical review. *Psychological Bulletin, 84*, 767-781.

This article reviews the different theories and treatment techniques available for bruxism. It can be obtained from Alan Glaros, 889 Bloomcrest, Bloomfield Hills, MI 48013.

Rosenbaum, M.S., & Allyon, T. (1981). Treating bruxism with the habit reversal technique. *Behavior Research and Therapy, 19*, 87-96.

This article gives an in-depth description of the habit reversal technique and describes why each phase of the technique is important. The article can be obtained from Michael Rosenbaum, 5904 Spanish Moss Ct., Mobile, AL 36609.

References

Cassisi, J., & McGlynn, F. (1988). Effects of EMG-activated alarms on nocturnal bruxism. *Behavior Therapy, 19*, 133-142.

Jenkins, J., & Peterson, G. (1978). Self-monitoring and self-administered aversion in the treatment of bruxism. *Journal of Behavior Therapy and Experimental Psychatry, 9*, 387-388.

Rosenbaum, M., & Allyon, T. (1981). Treating bruxism with the habit reversal technique. *Behavior Research and Therapy, 19*, 87-96.

8 Cancer

Assessment Strategies

The most emphasized problem area for behavioral intervention with cancer patients is conditioned nausea and vomiting resulting from chemotherapy treatment. For behavioral assessment, frequency counts and amount of time of nausea and vomiting can be recorded by the patient. Ratings of anxiety and nausea can be made at home before coming for treatment, waiting for treatment at the hospital, and during and after treatment. A seven point Likert-type scale, ranging from "not at all" to "extremely," can be used for these ratings.

Other areas that may require assessment include depression, pain, insomnia, and conversion disorders.

Treatment Strategies

The most commonly used behavioral treatment for conditioned nausea and vomiting associated with chemotherapy involves relaxation training and variants of relaxation training (e.g., guided imagery). Lyles, Burish, Krozely, and Oldham (1982) tell the patients that the goal of relaxation training is to become as calm and relaxed as possible during treatment, thus making the chemotherapy experience less unpleasant and reducing the probability and severity of side effects. Initial relaxation sessions can occur on days when no chemotherapy treatment is scheduled. Suggestions of calm in the absence of nausea can be integrated into the guided images. Relaxation training can then take place immediately before chemotherapy treatment sessions and continue throughout the actual treatments. The relaxation instructions can be continued for about five minutes after the completion of the chemotherapy in order to reduce the possibility of a conditioned response occuring to the completion of the treatment.

Live relaxation training during the treatments has been shown to be more effective than taped relaxation training (Morrow, 1984). Relaxation is also more effective if administered by a professional therapist rather than a volunteer (Carey & Burish, 1987). The session can be taped and the patient is instructed to practice the relaxation daily between sessions using the tape and imagining the chemotherapy session. Mastery of the relaxation procedure may allow the patient to use the skill, without the therapist's help, during the actual chemotherapy sessions. Therapist involvement during the chemotherapy sessions can be gradually faded out. Additionally, training the nurses who administer the chemotherapy in relaxation techniques may be helpful in transferring training from the therapist to the patient. Being able to use relaxation through recall and applying the relaxation skills to other anxiety producing situations may give the patient added confidence with the techniques.

The relaxation techniques are likely to be successful for the anticipatory nausea and for the chemically induced nausea. However, it is important to note that some of the post-chemotherapy side effects may be conditioned and are not due to the side effects of the medication. Systematic desensitization, using individualized hierarchies of the treatment procedure, has been found to be successful in one group study (Morrow & Morell, 1982).

Multiple site EMG biofeedback combined with relaxation training has also been effective in reducing the negative effects and conditioned nausea associated with chemotherapy treatment (Burish, Shartner, & Lyles, 1981).

Greene and Seime (1987) gave a patient a solution of equal parts of lemon juice and water during chemotherapy treatments to mask conditioned taste sensations. The treatment led to a decrease in anticipatory symptoms.

For More Information

Lyles, J., Burish, T., Krozely, M., & Oldham, R. (1982). Efficacy of relaxation training and guided imagery in reducing the aversiveness of cancer therapy. *Journal of Consulting and Clinical Psychology, 50*, 509-524.

This article reviews the previous research using relaxation training and similar approaches (e.g., hypnosis, biofeedback) to treat the conditioned nausea and vomiting associated with chemotherapy. The method of relaxation training and guided imagery is described. Suggestions are made for improving post-treatment response. The article can be obtained from Thomas G. Burish, Department of Psychology, Wesley Hall, Vanderbilt University, Nashville, TN 37240.

Redd, W., & Andrykowski, M. (1982). Behavioral intervention in cancer treatment: Controlling aversion reactions to chemotherapy. *Journal of Consulting and Clinical Psychology, 50*, 1018-1029.

This article reviews the toxic effects of chemotherapy and the different methods used for controlling chemotherapy nausea and emesis. Included is a discussion of assessment and clinical issues. The article can be obtained from Dr. William Redd, Psychology Department, 603 E. Daniel, University of Illinois, Champaign, IL 61820.

References

Burish, T., Shartner, C., & Lyles, J. (1981). Effectiveness of multiple muscle-site EMG biofeedback and relaxation training in reducing the aversiveness of cancer chemotherapy. *Biofeedback and Self-Regulation, 6*, 523-535.

Carey, M., & Burish, T. (1987). Providing relaxation training to cancer chemotherapy patients: A comparison of three delivery techniques. *Journal of Consulting and Clinical Psychology, 55*, 732-737.

Greene, P., & Seime, R. (1987). Stimulus control of anticipatory nausea in a cancer chemotherapy. *Journal of Behavior Therapy and Experimental Psychiatry, 18*, 61-64.

Lyles, J., Burish, T., Krozely, M., & Oldham, R. (1982). Efficacy of relaxation training and guided imagery in reducing the aversiveness of cancer chemotherapy. *Journal of Consulting and Clinical Psychology, 50*, 509-524.

Morrow, G. (1984). Appropriateness of taped versus live relaxation in the systematic desensitization of anticipatory nausea and vomiting in cancer patients. *Journal of Consulting and Clinical Psychology, 52*, 1098-1099.

Morrow, G., & Morrell, C. (1982). *The antiemetic efficacy of behavioral treatment for cancer chemotherapy induced anticipatory nausea and vomiting: A randomized trial of systematic desensitization, counseling placebo and no treatment.* Unpublished manuscript.

See Also

Chapter 29. Pain - Acute
Chapter 40. Vomiting

9 Colitis

Assessment Strategies

There are two basic forms of colitis: ulcerative and spastic. Ulcerative colitis is a persistent and chronic inflammation of the colon with bloody diarrhea. Spastic or mucous colitis affects the motor activity and mucous secreting functions of the colon. The diagnosis of either type of colitis should be confirmed by a physician before any behavioral assessment is initiated. Behavioral assessment involves keeping a daily record of the frequency of colitis attacks. A colitis attack usually involves abdominal cramping and diarrhea. A behavioral diary containing both the behavioral and cognitive antecedents to an attack and a 1 to 10 rating of muscle tension will also be helpful.

Treatment Strategies

Stress is the most commonly reported antecedent to colitis attacks. Successful management of colitis attacks uses relaxation training and self-control procedures (e.g., Mitchell, 1978; Youell & McCollough, 1975). Relaxation training should emphasize abdominal relaxation and the reduction of pre-attack tension. The beginning of any pain should serve as a stimulus for using the relaxation techniques.

Self-control techniques that have been utilized successfully include: 1) thought stopping and worry time to manage thoughts, and 2) self-desensitization and cognitive restructuring to manage any fears. This type of program can be successfully completed within 20 weekly sessions.

For More Information *and* References

Mitchell, K. (1978). Self-management of spastic colitis. *Journal of Behavior Therapy and Experimental Psychiatry, 9*, 269-272.

This article describes the different types of colitis and the use of self-management, including relaxation training, in a single study. The article can be obtained from Kenneth R. Mitchell, Division of Developmental and Social Medicine, Faculty of Madison, University of New Castle, 2308, Australia.

Youell, K., & McCullough, J. (1975). Behavioral treatment of mucous colitis. *Journal of Consulting and Clinical Psychology, 5*,740-745.

This case study emphasizes the use of cognitive restructuring as a coping strategy for colitis attacks. The article can be obtained from James P. McCullough, Virginia Commonwealth University, Psychological Service Center, 800 West Franklin Street, Richmond, VA 23284.

See Also

Chapter 12. Conversion Disorders

10 Compliance

Assessment Strategies

Shelton and Levy (1981) define compliance as "carrying out an assignment in the way described by the assignment giver(s) . . . at the time, in the place, and in the manner presented" (p. 37). This chapter will focus on compliance related to appointment keeping, medication taking, and following behavioral assignments used in the course of treating other problems (e.g., recording daily food intake for the treatment of anorexia).

Behavioral assessment of compliance can be obtained by direct observation, patient's self-report, or report by significant others. Appointment keeping is best assessed by direct observation. Frankel and Hovell (1978) believe the best formula for determining an overall index of appointment keeping is the "sum of each client's proportion of kept appointments per time period to the total number of clients for this time period" (p. 443).

Medication taking can be assessed by directly observing the patient take pills, by patient's self-report (although self-report tends to overestimate compliance), or by monitoring the amount of medication remaining. It can also be assessed by the use of a chemical marker in the drug that is excreted through the patient's urine. The fact that a patient improves may also be an indication of compliance with medication. For example, if a patient takes medication for hypertension, blood pressure should be lowered.

A functional analysis of compliance may be helpful. Zifferblatt (1975) used a behavioral log to assess medication compliance. The log consisted of the following categories: date, time, antecedents (cues and people), consequences, and relevant thoughts.

A variation of patient's self-report involves having the patient contact the therapist on a regular basis to report his or her adherence to a treatment plan. Hammonds and Worthington (1982) required that patients telephone the therapist with data on performance. They describe this procedure as follows:

> **Each night three and one-half hours were designated as call-in times, during which participants . . . phoned in data for the preceding 24 hours. Data were recorded on an automatic telephone answering system and participants had no nightly personal contact with the therapist. Frequency of prescribed call-in was a behavioral measure of compliance. The self-reported phoned-in data, e.g., number of calories consumed and duration of exercise, provided the second type of compliance measure. If participants failed to call in, they called in the following night and reported data for both nights. [p. 5]**

Treatment Strategies

In general, it has been found that non-compliance increases with the complexity of the assignment. In some cases, simply educating the patient about the problem of non-compliance is successful in increasing compliance. Walker (1981) found that teaching patients about the importance of taking lithium regularly served to increase compliance. However, Haynes et al. (1981) found that education was not effective in increasing medication compliance with hypertensive patients.

Stimulus control techniques may be effective in improving compliance related to keeping appointments. Both postcard reminders and telephone calls have been used as antecedent cues (Gates & Colborn, 1976; Schroeder, 1973; Shepad & Moseley, 1976). Postcards tend to be more cost-effective and need only state the date, time, and place of appointment. These reminders generally are used three to seven days prior to the scheduled appointment. However, the use of these cues may not be effective in some settings (Barkin & Duncan, 1975; Kidd & Euphrat, 1971).

Cues and prompts have also been found to be effective in improving compliance in taking medication. Pill "calendars" can include a prepackaged daily dose of a patient's medication stapled to each day on the calendar (Moulding, 1961). Timed buzzers or signals have been used as prompts to take medication. Medication taking can also be cued to a patient's daily routine (Haynes et al., 1976).

For behavioral assignments, specific written instructions may act as a cue to comply. In addition, phone calls placed by the therapist and prompts from significant others in the patient's environment may aid in increasing compliance. Grady (1984) used calendars with reminder stickers and postcard reminders to significantly improve compliance with breast self-exams.

Meyers, Thackwray, Johnson, and Schleser (1983) found that a combination of stimulus control techniques, including postcards, telephone calls, and home visits, was more effective in increasing appointment compliance than use of any one of these techniques alone.

Some behaviors consequent to medication taking will aid in improving future medication taking. For example, the patient could replace the medication in an observable and prominent location after use.

Self-monitoring is successful in increasing compliance in some cases. Epstein and Masek (1978) had students record on data sheets the time that they took vitamin C. This simple self-monitoring improved compliance. Specific training in self-monitoring maybe more effective than simply giving instructions to the patient.

A verbal or written commitment obtained from the patient may improve compliance for some behaviors. Wurtele, Galanos, and Roberts (1980) found this effective in ensuring that persons returned for a TB test. However, it may not be effective in more complex tasks, such as appointment keeping in a general medicine clinic (Levy & Clark, 1980).

Contingency contracts have been used with success in increasing all types of compliance. Shelton and Levy (1981) list the basic rules for developing a contingency contract to be used in improving compliance with homework assignments as follows:

1. **A very clear and detailed description of the homework should be stated.**
2. **The contract should specify the positive reinforcements gained if the homework is completed.**
3. **Some provision should be made for some consequence for failure to complete the behavioral assignment within a specified time limit or behavior frequency.**

> 4. **The contract should specify the means by which the contracted response is to be observed, measured, and recorded.**
> 5. **An arrangement should be made so that the timing for delivery of reinforcement contingencies follows the response as quickly as possible. [p. 48]**

The contracts are usually written, dated, and signed, and the rewards contained in the contract are often negotiated between the therapist, the patient, and/or significant other. An example of this type of contract for a chronic pain patient follows:

> **I agree to do my assigned homework involving (1) walking every morning twice around my block; (2) doing 15 sit-ups; (3) taking the pain cocktail before going to sleep at night; and (4) getting out of the house at least once per day for a half hour or more. Harold (my husband) will monitor my progress and report it to Dr. Shelton on Mondays and Thursdays. The reward for completing all homework as assigned will involve a choice of the following:**
>
> **A. Attending a movie**
> **B. Riding in the car for a short drive**
> **C. Having Harold join me for TV**
> **D. Having Harold give me a back rub**
>
> **I get one of these rewards for each day that I complete my homework assignment. This contract will be renegotiated and new homework added in 2 weeks during my next scheduled appointment.**
>
> **Signature__________________________**
>
> **Signature__________________________**
>
> **[Shelton & Levy, 1981; p. 49]**

Specific behaviors are often shaped gradually. Monetary contingencies are often included in these contracts. This may involve forfeiture of a certain amount of money if the patient misses a scheduled session and a refund of money contingent on attendance. Money can also be lost if the patient does not complete certain assignments and can be refunded upon successful completion. Another reward commonly used in contracts is additional therapy time.

Zeisat (1982) believes that the therapist should provide the patient with the rationale for the contract.

> **It should be stressed that the contract represents a concrete commitment on the part of both parties concerned, so that both doctor and patient have certain obligations to each other in working on the patient's problem. The patient should understand that it is expected that, once he agrees to this contract, he will abide by it, although discussions may occur periodically to reevaluate the program and to make appropriate modifications. [p. 276]**

If the behavior to be shaped is a new skill for the patient, the in-session use of such techniques as modeling, coaching, prompting, and rehearsal may be necessary to ensure successful completion of the assignment by the patient.

Cognitive techniques can be useful in dealing with non-compliance. Some patients may have cognitions that interfere with completion of an assignment. The use of a cognitive technique such as Self-Instructional Training helps the patient in preparing cognitively for an assignment, confronting the assignment, and self-reinforcing for the completion of the assignment. Cochran (1984) successfully used a six-week cognitive-behavioral intervention, similar to Beck's, to improve compliance in taking lithium among manic-depressive patients.

Family involvement may also aid in compliance. Family members can be instructed in reinforcing compliance and withdrawing reinforcement when the patient is non-compliant. For some problems pairing the patient with a family member or with another patient with a similar problem may improve compliance with assignments.

For More Information

Frankel, B., & Hovell, M. (1978). Health service appointment keeping. A behavioral view and critical review. *Behavior Modification, 2*, 435-464.

This article reviews the behavioral assessment and treatment of compliance with appointment keeping. Antecedent cues and appointment consequences are discussed. The article can be obtained from Melvourne Hovell, Health Promotion, School of Public Health, SDSH, San Diego, CA 92182.

Shelton, J., & Levy, R. (1981). *Behavioral assignments and treatment compliance: A handbook of clinical strategies.* Champaign, IL: Research Press.

This book reviews the use of behavioral assignments in clinical practice and contains numerous techniques for enhancing compliance with behavioral assignments. Behavioral assignments and compliance are discussed specifically for the following problems: anxiety, depression, marital problems, addictive behaviors, obesity, chronic operant pain, sexual dysfunction, shyness, non-assertion, and parenting skills. The book can be obtained from Research Press, 2612 N. Mattis Avenue, Champaign, IL 61820.

Ziesat, G, (1982). Adhering to medical regimen. in P. Boudewyns and F. Keefe (Eds.), *Behavioral Medicine in General Medicine Practice* (pp. 269-294). Reading, MA: Addison-Wesley.

This chapter reviews the different assessment methods of non-compliance, including: pill counts, chemical markers, improved health and recordkeeping by the patient. The therapeutic techniques of behavioral contracting, monitoring, stimulus control, operant conditioning procedures, and cognitive methods are reviewed. A case study is included. The book can be obtained from Addison-Wesley Publishing Company, 1 Jacob Way, Reading, MA 01867.

Zifferblatt, S. (1975). Increasing patient compliance through the applied analysis of behavior. *Preventative Medicine, 4*, 173-182.

This article describes how the applied analysis of behavior can be used to increase patient compliance. Specific examples regarding compliance with medication taking are included. The article can be obtained from Steven Zifferblatt, Ph.D., 3815 Mainsail Circle, Westlake Village, CA 91361.

References

Barkin, R., & Duncan, B. (1975). Broken appointments: questions, not answers. *Pediatrics, 55*, 747-748.

Cochran, S. (1984). Preventing medical non-compliance in the outpatient treatment of bipolar affective disorders. *Journal of Consulting and Clinical Psychology, 52*, 873-878.

Epstein, L., & Masek, B. (1978). Behavioral control of medicine compliance. *Journal of Applied Behavior Analysis, 11*, 1-9.

Frankel, B., & Hovell, M. (1978). Health service appointment keeping. A behavioral view and critical review. *Behavior Modification, 2*, 435-464.

Gates, S., & Colborn, K. (1976). Lowering appointment failures in a neighborhood health center. *Medical Care, 14*, 263-267.

Grady, K. (1984). Cue enhancement in the long-term practice of breast self-examination. *Journal of Behavioral Medicine, 7*, 191-204.

Haynes, R., Sackett, D., Gibson, E., Taylor, D., Hackett, B., Roberts, R., & Johnson, A. (1976). Improvement of medication compliance in uncontrolled hypertension. *The Lancet, 1*, 1265-1268.

Hammonds, T., & Worthington, E. (1982, August). *Compliance with homework tasks in a behavioral self-control weight loss program.* Paper presented at the meeting of the American Psychological Association, Washington, D.C.

Kidd, A., & Euphrat, J. (1971). Why prospective outpatients fail to make or keep appointments. *Journal of Clinical Psychology, 27*, 394-395.

Levy, R., & Clark, H. (1980). The use of an overt commitment to enhance compliance: a cautionary note. *Journal of Behavior Therapy and Experimental Psychiatry, 11*, 105-107.

Meyers, A.W., Thackway, D.E., Johnson, C.B., & Schleser, R. (1983). A comparison of prompting strategies for improving appointment compliance of hypertensive individuals. *Behavior Therapy, 14*, 267-274.

Moulding, T. (1961). Preliminary study of the pill calendar as a method of improving the self-administration of drugs. *American Review of Respiratory Disorders, 84*, 284-287.

Sackett, D., Haynes, R., Gibson, E., Hackett, B., Taylor, D., Roberts, R., & Johnson, A. (1975). Randomized clinical trial of strategies for improving medication compliance in primary hypertension. *The Lancet, 1*, 1205-1207.

Shelton, J., & Levy, R. (1981). *Behavioral assignments and treatment compliance: A handbook of clinical strategies.* Champaign, IL: Research Press.

Shepard, D., & Moseley, T. (1976). Mailed vs. telephoned appointment reminders to reduce broken appointments in a hospital outpatient department. *Medical Care, 14*, 268-273.

Walker, J. (1981). Use of a patient education booklet to improve compliance with lithium therapy. *Psychosomatics, 22*, 51.

Wurtele, S., Galanos, A., & Roberts, M. (1980). Increasing return compliance in a tuberculosis detection drive. *Journal of Behavioral Medicine, 3*, 311-318.

Ziesat, H. (1982). Adhering to medical regimen. In P. Boudewyns & F. Keefe (Eds.), *Behavioral medicine in general medicine practice* (pp.269-294). Reading, MA: Addison-Wesley.

Zifferblatt, S. (1975). Increasing patient compliance through the applied analysis of behavior. *Preventative Medicine, 4*, 173-182.

11 Constipation

Assessment Strategies

A physical exam is necessary to rule out organic causes of the constipation. McCubbin, Surwit, and Marsbach (1987) have utilized a rectal balloon assembly (Arndorfer Medical Specialties, Greendale, WI) to assess sphincter reflexes and rectal sensations. Behavioral assessment should consist of a two-week baseline period to determine the number of spontaneous eliminations. The date and time of day should be recorded for each instance. The patient should be encouraged not to take laxatives during this baseline period.

Treatment Strategies

A classical conditioning model has been successful in treating constipation (Rovetto, 1979). Patients are told that regular evacuation is "dependent on conditioning to a specific date or set of habits" (p. 144). The conditioning sequence includes the use of a glycerin suppository along with morning coffee and reading a newspaper or a book. The suggested sequence is coffee, then suppository, then reading, then elimination. Learning can be enhanced by instructing the patient to take a mild laxative after each meal. Twelve consecutive conditioning days are suggested. Additionally, booster treatments may be scheduled to avoid extinction.

McCubbin et al. (1987) successfully employed a marometrically based sensory discrimination procedure utilizing a rectal balloon to reduce the sensory threshold for rectal distention for one patient. The discrimination procedure utilizes shaping with immediate feedback and positive reinforcement.

For More Information

Rovetto, F. (1979). Treatment of chronic constipation by classical conditioning techniques. *Journal of Behavior Therapy and Experimental Psychiatry, 10*, 143-146.

This article describes in detail a classical conditioning technique used to treat constipation in eight adult female patients. The article can be obtained from Francesco Rovetto, Professore Incaricato, Instituto di Psicologia, Facolta di Medicina e Chirurgia, Universite Statele, Via F. Stoiza 23, Milano, Italy.

References

McCubbin, J.J., Surwit, R., & Marsbach, C. (1987). Sensory discrimination in the treatment of a case of chronic constipation. *Behavior Therapy, 18*, 273-278.

Rovetto, F. (1979). Treatment of chronic constipation by classical conditioning techniques. *Journal of Behavior Therapy and Experimental Psychiatry, 10*, 143-146.

12 Conversion Disorders[1]

Assessment Strategies

Conversion disorders (hysterical reactions) are characterized by discrete pseudoneurological symptoms such as blindness, deafness, aphonia, and astasia-abasia. A thorough medical evaluation is necessary to distinguish these disorders from true physical disorders. In many cases, specific medical specialists or examinations (e.g., an ophthalmologist to test for hysterical blindness or a laryngoscopic exam for aphonia) will be needed for a complete medical evaluation.

In general, behavioral assessment of conversion disorders involves the recording of frequency, the intensity of specific symptoms, the adaptive behaviors which may be currently occuring at a very low rate, or all three. Examples of behavioral assessment include: number of daily episodes of psychogenic vomiting and amount of distance walked for a patient with hysterical leg weakness. It may also be important to note if the symptom occurs more frequently in certain settings or in the presence of particular individuals.

For some conversion disorders (e.g., total hysterical blindness or deafness) it may not be possible to conduct any behavioral assessment.

Treatment Strategies

Most conversion disorders can be treated with a combination of extinction and reinforcement techniques. The techniques can easily be applied on a medical ward if necessary. Extinction programs are especially effective for patients who obtain any reinforcement from their symptoms. Reinforcement may be monetary compensation or simply the attention or concern of others. Patients may initially be told that their physical problems have no organic basis. Instructions can then be given to the hospital staff, the patient's family, and friends to ignore the patient whenever the symptoms are evident or when the patient complains of the symptoms. In a hospital, a period of time out can also be used whenever the patient complains of the symptoms. Cautela (1971) has also demonstrated the successful use of covert extinction. In covert extinction, the patient imagines the removal of the rewards he or she currently receives for the physical symptoms.

If patients appear to be receiving reinforcement from the comforts of the hospital, it may also be necessary to remove some of the reinforcement of the hospital environment. For example, it may be necessary to place the patient in a very dull-looking room.

Reinforcement of adaptive, "healthy behaviors" can be used for every patient displaying conversion symptoms. The most commonly used reinforcers are simple verbal praise, attention, and smiling. Agras, Leitenberg, Barlow, and Thompson (1969) describe a reinforcement program for astasia-abasia patients:

---

[1]The many different conversion disorder symptoms discussed in this chapter can generally be treated with similar techniques.

"Reinforcement consisted of praise such as `good . . . excellent . . . that's a good one' for good steps, and of two minutes conversation with the therapist when she met the reinforcement criterion for distance walked. This criterion was established as the mean between the previous criterion and the next highest trial" (p. 1436). Other material rewards can also be used if necessary.

Some behaviors, such as walking, may have to be shaped gradually. Any behavior incompatible with somatic complaints should also be reinforced. Examples include; physical and recreational activity and social interactions. Patients can be asked to display their progress graphically. As with the extinction programs, family and friends should be instructed on the use of reinforcement techniques. Some innovative conditioning techniques have been used to treat hysterical blindness and deafness. Parry-Jones, Santer-Westrate, and Crawley (1969) describe the following procedure for treating hysterical blindness:

> **The patient was required to press a button at intervals of 20 sec. A response which followed the preceding one within 18-21 sec. would be marked, and hence reinforced, by the sounding of a buzzer. Responses occurring at less than 18 or more than 21 sec. would not be reinforced, i.e., no buzzer would sound, and the apparatus would reset itself immediately. After the patient's performance was stabilized, visual stimuli were introduced which could serve as cues for correct spacing of responses, i.e., a light bulb would flash on every 18-21 sec. The patient could now improve her performance by making use of these visual cues. [p. 81]**

Once the patient is able to see the light on every occasion, the intensity of the light may be reduced.

Malmo, Davis, and Barza (1952) used a procedure to rapidly treat hysterical deafness that involves conditioning a patient by using shock. Instructions given to the patient were as follows:

> **You are to sit on this chair as comfortably as you can and place your right middle finger on this button, with the underpart, not the end of the finger, in contact with the silver electrode. . . . When the shock comes, lift your finger and put it right down again, because the shock will be over very quickly. . . . The next thing I am going to do is sound a tone from the other room just to see if it is working properly. During the session, this tone will sound before every shock. Now if your finger should tend to lift up just before the shock comes along, don't worry about it—just let it come up, and then put it right down again. [p. 195]**

In dealing with hysterical aphonia, it is suggested that a speech therapist be used for the voice retraining. Speech can be shaped in one session, starting with the patient humming or coughing.

Walton and Black (1959) combined a reward and punishment procedure to successfully treat hysterical aphonia. They describe the procedure as follows:

> **M. was required to read from a book into the microphone of a tape recorder. The book chosen was judged by two psychologists concerned to be basically uninteresting to M. The explanation given was that: "Her voice needed systematic exercise and that this could be achieved by her reading, or trying to read, aloud from the chosen book for periods of 15 min at a time. The volume of her voice would then be measured from the tape recording. If she fails to either maintain the volume of her speech throughout the 15 min or to improve the volume on successive 15 min**

sessions then it would be evident that she was in need of more extensive exercise. An extra 2 min would be added on each session, in these circumstances, until improvement was made, when the session would be judged to have attained an optimum length for the most beneficial effects of the exercise to be felt. If, on the other hand, improvement were made within a 15 min session, or from one session to the next, then the exercises must be having effect. In order to avoid excessive fatigue, sessions would then be reduced by 2 min so long as improvement was maintained." [p. 305]

Relaxation training can useful for conversion disorders involving muscle tenseness (e.g., tight throat and larynx muscles involved in aphonia). Assertive training can be helpful for some patients who exhibit conversion disorders when taught new methods of searching for and obtaining attention from the environment. Stress management techniques may also be used to teach patients alternative coping strategies for stressful situations.

Some hysterical reactions contain strong phobic elements (e.g., hyperesthesia of taste). For these patients the use of systematic desensitization may be helpful. Beyme (1964) used stimuli that could reciprocally inhibit the conditioned reactions (e.g., sugar for an acid taste and soothing ointment for unpleasant sensations of touch.) For example, "After imagining an orange slice had elicited a distinct increase in the flow of saliva in the relaxed patient, he took a very small bit of sugar into his mouth, about one-eighth of the size of an ordinary lump of sugar. Immediately afterwards, he was again asked to imagine an orange slice. He could now notice no reaction" (p. 9). Additionally, if stress producing situations elicit the hysterical reaction, the patient may need to be desensitized to the situations.

Direct punishment of the hysterical behaviors has not proved to be an effective long-term treatment (Singh, 1975).

For More Information

Bird, J. (1979). Behavioral treatment of hysteria. *British Journal of Psychiatry, 134*, 129-137.

This article presents a good defintion of conversion disorders and reviews the common behavioral treatments for conversion disorders. The article can be obtained from Julian Bird, Senior Registrar, The Maudsley Hospital, Denmark Hill, London, SE 5, England.

Blanchard, E., & Hersen, M. (1976). Behavioral treatment of hysterical neurosis: Symptom substitution and symptom return reconsidered. *Psychiatry, 39*, 118-129.

This article reviews the theoretical model of neurotic disorders in general and presents 3 adult case studies demonstrating the techniques of extinction, reinforcement, and assertion training with different conversion symptoms. The issue of symptom substitution is also discussed. The article can be obtained from Edward Blanchard, Department of Psychology, SUNY at Albany, New York 12222.

Meichenbaum, D. (1966). Sequential strategies in two cases of hysteria. *Behavior Research and Therapy, 4*, 89-94.

This article describes the successful use of relaxation, systematic desensitization, and assertion training with a patient who is unable to keep his eyes open, and the successful use of extinction and reinforcement with a patient displaying hysterical leg paralysis. The article can be obtained from Donald Michenbaum, Department of Psychology, University of Waterloo, Waterloo, Ontario N2L 3G1 Canada.

References

Agras, S., Leitenberg, H., Barlow, D., & Thomson, E. (1969). Instructions and reinforcement in the modification of neurotic behavior. *American Journal of Psychiatry, 125*, 1335-1439.

Beyme, F. (1964). Hyperesthesia of taste and touch treated by reciprocal inhibition. *Behavior Research and Therapy, 2*, 7-14.

Cautela, J. (1971). Covert extinction. *Behavior Therapy, 2*, 192-200.

Malmo, R., Davis, J., & Barza, S. (1952). Total hysterical deafness: An experimental case study. *Journal of Personality, 21*, 188-304.

Parry-Jones, W., Santer-Westrate, H., & Crawley, R. (1970). Behavior therapy in a case of hysterical blindness. *Behavior Research and Therapy, 8*, 79-85.

Singh, R. (1975). Experiments in two cases of hysterical fits. *Journal of Behavior Therapy and Experimental Psychiatry, 6* , 351-353.

Walton, D., & Black, D. (1959). The application of modern learning theory treatment of chronic hysterical aphonia. *Journal of Psychosomatic Research, 3*, 303-311.

13 Dental Fear

Assessment Strategies

Many different factors contribute to dental fear. A patient may have anxiety about the anticipated pain, the anesthetic injection, the sounds and smells of the dental office, or anticipated criticism about his poor oral hygeine, or all of these. Vrand, McNeil, and McGlynn (1986) have developed an 11-item structured interview form for assessing dental fear.

Self-report measures may be helpful for assessment and monitoring of progress during treatment. One commonly used scale is the Dental Anxiety Scale (Corah, 1969) (see Figure 13-1).

The Dental Fear Survey (Kleinknecht, Klepac, & Alexander, 1973; Figure 13-2) is another useful self-report inventory for creating a hierarchy during treatment.

The State-Trait Anxiety Inventory (Spielberger, Gorsuch, & Lushene) may also be used to discriminate the patient's anxiety during dental treatment from the general level of anxiety.

One of the simplest assessments is to conduct a behavioral avoidance test to determine how far the patient can go in actually completing dental work. Patients can be instructed to attempt each of the steps (9-19) on the Dental Fear Survey, and rate their fear of each step in the process on a 0-to-100 SUDS scale (see chapter ??).

The patient can also rate any expected, or any experienced, pain during each step. If the patient is able to reach the twelfth step of the hierarchy, sitting in the dental chair, it is also possible to have the dentist rate the patient's overt anxiety on such variables as movement in the chair, head movements, and overall tension.

Figure 16-1

DENTAL ANXIETY SCALE

1. If you had to go the the dentist tomorrow, how would you feel about it?

a) I would look forward to it as a reasonably enjoyable experience. b) I wouldn't care one way or the other. c) I would be a little uneasy about it. d) I would be afraid that it would be unpleasant and painful. e) I would be very frightened of what the dentist might do.

2. When you are waiting in the dentist's office for your turn in the chair, how do you feel?

a) Relaxed. b) A little uneasy. c) Tense. d) Anxious. e) So anxious that I sometimes break out in a sweat or almost feel physically sick.

3. When you are in the dentist's chair waiting while he gets his drill ready to begin working on your teeth, how do you feel? (Same alternatives as number 2).

4. You are in the dentist's chair to have your teeth cleaned. While you are waiting and the dentist is getting out the instruments which he will use to scrape your teeth around the gums, how do you feel? (Same alternatives as number 2).

[Corah, 1969, p. 596]

Figure 16-2

DENTAL FEAR SURVEY

Item

Avoidance of dentistry	**(1, never - 5, often)**
1. Have avoided calling for appointment	
2. Have canceled or not appeared	
Felt physiological responses	**(1, none - 5, great)**
3. Muscles become tense	
4. Breathing increases	
5. Perspiration increases	
6. Nausea	
7. Heart rate increases	
8. Mouth salivates	
Fearfulness of stimuli	**(1, none - 5, great)**
9. Making an appointment	
10. Approaching office	
11. Waiting room	
12. Dental chair	
13. Smell of office	
14. Seeing dentist	
15. Seeing needle	
16. Feeling needle	
17. Seeing drill	
18. Hearing drill	
19. Feeling drill	
20. Feeling as if you will gag	
21. Having teeth cleaned	
22. Feeling pain even after anesthetic injection	
23. Generally how fearful are you of dentistry	
How fearful were your:	
24. Mother	
25. Father	
26. Brothers and sisters	
27. Childhood friends	

Treatment Strategies

A number of effective strategies have been employed to treat dental fears. Auerbach, Kendall, Cuttler, and Levitt (1976) found that providing individuals who have an internal locus of control, with specific information about the dental procedures and expected sensations, reduced dental anxiety. However, individuals with an external locus of control responded better to information containing generalities about the dental clinics, staff, and procedures.

Desensitization, both in vivo and in vitro, has been found to be very effective in treating dental fears (Gale & Ayer, 1969). A sample hierarchy is shown in Figure 13-3.

Figure 13-3

HIERARCHY FOR SYSTEMATIC DESENSITIZATION

1. Thinking about going to the dentist.
2. Getting in your car to go to the dentist.
3. Calling for an appointment with the dentist.
4. Sitting in the waiting room of the dentist's office.
5. Having the nurse tell you it's your turn.
6. Getting in the dentist's chair.
7. Seeing the dentist lay out his instruments, one of which is a probe.
8. Having a probe held in front of you while you look at it.
9. Having a probe placed on the side of a tooth.
10. Having a probe placed in a cavity.
11. Getting an injection in your gums on one side.
12. Having your teeth drilled and worrying that the anesthetic will wear off.
13. Getting two injections, one on each side.

[Gale & Ayer, 1969, p. 1306]

For some patients the relaxation training alone (progressive muscle relaxation or cue-controlled relaxation) is all that is needed (Beck, Karl, & Russell, 1978; Miller, Murphy, & Miller, 1978). Jerremalm, Jansson, and Ost (1986) describe an applied relaxation program for dental fear as follows:

> **The relaxation training was started with tension-release of the muscles. The muscle groups of the body were divided into two parts introduced during Sessions 2 and 3. Session 4 introduced a release-only version. During the 5th session a cue-controlled relaxation was introduced and personal positive scenes were developed to be used as a coping alternative to the usual release of bodily tension during more painful dental restorations. Homework assignments were relaxation training on a daily basis, self-monitoring of bodily reactions to dental stimuli and readings of relevant material during treatment. Session 7 was devoted to training in differential relaxation and to the rehearsal of images of the positive scene. During Sessions 7 and 8 the application training was done through a graded approach to the dentist's office: in Session 7 listening to an audio recording of a real dental restoration and in Session 8 entering a dentist's office with the therapist and the entire group of 4 patients. During Session 9 treatment was summed up, repeating self- instructions, preparing for the first visit to a dentist soon after treatment. If necessary therapists could accompany the patients on their first visits to the dentist. Patients were provided with written material to be presented to the dentist describing both the treatment for the dental fear and ways the dentist could be helpful making them feel comfortable and introduce the procedures in a smooth and stepwise fashion. [p. 590]**

Corah, Gale, and Illia (1979) have used relaxation training presented through headphones during dental treatment. They describe the procedure as follows: "The instructions stress the relaxation of various muscle groups with the exception of the jaw muscles. The presentation was begun three to four minutes before the dentist administered anesthesia and continued until the dental procedure was completed" (p. 1348). Symbolic, or participant, modeling has also been found to be effective (Bernstein & Kleinknecht, 1982). Kleinknecht and Bernstein (1979) describe the symbolic modeling procedure as follows:

> **Clients viewed a 20-min. videotape in which a patient (model) telephones a dentist for an appointment, drives to the office, sits in the waiting room, and then undergoes an oral examination. During the examination the dentist finds a cavity which he offers to fill. The patient reluctantly agrees and the procedure is carried out. The model displays initial apprehension, but with reassurance by the dentist, and through verbalized attempts to demonstrate self-control over the situation, becomes more relaxed and confident. Two versions of the tape were shown, one with a female and one with a male model. Clients were instructed to observe the model, to be aware of the physical and cognitive reactions experienced, and to relax when needed. [p. 311]**

Flooding has been used less frequently but has also been shown to be effective. Mathews and Rezin (1977) used four different realistic dental themes, each lasting about 12 minutes, (e.g., acute toothache requiring an extraction). The combination of modeling, graduated exposure, and self-paced practice has proven to be an effective treatment package.

Kleinknecht and Bernstein (1979) describe the graduated exposure and self-paced practice:

> **Graduated exposure presented hierarchically arranged, ten-second videotaped segments of a dental procedure, as viewed from the patient's perspective. The clients viewed these segments while in a relatively relaxed state brought about by therapist guided relaxation instructions. This procedure was carried out in a manner similar to systematic desensitization in that, if anxiety was experienced, the scene was terminated until the client became relaxed again. Progress to the next item on the hierarchy occurred when the client could view two consecutive presentations of a given segment while remaining relaxed. In the self-paced practice component of treatment, the clients were aided in setting up a convenient time to simply sit in the waiting room of a cooperating dentist. They were told to relax and attend to the sights and sounds of the office. Following the waiting room experience, clients scheduled a time (e.g., at lunch or between regular dental patients) to explore the dental operatory equipment (including the handpiece, or drill) and relax in the dental chair. A dental assistant was present to demonstrate various pieces of equipment and explain their function. [pp. 311-312]**

Jerremalm et al. (1986) used self-instructional training to successfully reduce dental anxiety. They describe the procedure as follows:

> **The focus for the SIT treatment was on the negative thoughts confronted in the different phases of the dental contact. Patients were asked to record negative thoughts that were part of, and which augmented their fear of dentistry both before and during oral examinations and restorations. During treatment they were taught to produce a new rationale and calming self-instructions regarding what happened, to be used in each phase of the contact. Each patient was encouraged to produce his/her personally effective instructions, based upon previous successfully undertaken copings with different situations other than the dental fear situations. . . patients spent time developing a personal set of images, scenes to think about during phases of the dental treatment contact that were assumed to be extra hard to go through. These images and self-instructions were rehearsed both during sessions and as homework assignments. [pp. 590-591]**

Moses and Hollandsworth (1985) used a one-session (3 1/2 hour) stress inoculation package that included a description of the pain experience, training in coping skills, and exposure to a muscle pain task. The techniques were successful in enabling patients with a dental phobia to follow through with a dental appointment.

Klepac, Hauge, and Dowling (1982) successfully treated a patient whose overactive gag reflex interfered with dental treatment. They first taught the patient relaxation, with an emphasis on the muscles of the tongue and throat. Then the patient was taught to swallow with his mouth open. The coping skills of breathing, relaxation, and positive self-statements were also incorporated into the treatment program.

Frontalis EMG biofeedback with the patient in a dental chair has also been found effective in treating dental anxiety (Miller, Murphy, & Miller, 1978). Klepac (1975) devised a procedure for increasing pain tolerance by use of electric shock.

For More Information

Bernstein, D., & Kleinknecht, R. (1982). Multiple approaches to the reduction of dental fear. *Journal of Behavior Therapy and Experimental Psychiatry, 13*, 287-292.

This article compares the techniques of graduated exposure, participant modeling, and symbolic modeling for the treatment of dental fear. Included is a good description of each technique. The article can be obtained from Douglas Bernstein, Department of Psychology, University of Illinois, 603 East Daniel, Champaign, IL 61820.

Kleinknecht, R., & Bernstein, D. (1979). Short term treatment of dental avoidance. *Journal of Behavior Therapy and Experimental Psychiatry, 10*, 311-315.

This article describes the combined treatment of symbolic modeling, graduated exposure, and self-paced practice with three patients who exhibited dental fear. The article can be obtained from Ronald Kleinknecht, Western Washington University, Bellingham, WA 98225.

Melamed, B. (1979). Behavioral approaches to fear in dental settings. In M. Hersen, R. Eisler, & P. Miller (Eds.), *Progress in Behavior Modification* (pp. 171-203), *7*, New York: Academic Press.

This article reviews the different assessment techniques and behavioral approaches to dental fear. Included is a review of systematic desensitization and modeling studies with both adults and children. The book can be obtained from Academic Press, 111 Fifth Avenue, New York, NY 10003 or 6277 Sea Harbor Drive, Orlando, FL 32821.

References

Auerbach, S., Kendall, P., Cuttler, H., & Levitt, N. (1976). Anxiety, locus of control, type of preparatory information and adjustment to dental surgery.

Journal of Consulting and Clinical Psychology, 44, 809-818.

Beck, F., Karl, T., & Russell, R. (1978). Treatment of dental anxiety by cue-controlled relaxation. *Journal of Counseling Psychology, 25*, 591-594.

Bernstein, D., & Kleinknecht, R. (1982). Multiple approaches to the reduction of dental fear. *Journal of Behavior Therapy and Experimental Psychiatry, 13*, 287-292.

Corah, N. (1969). Development of a dental anxiety scale. *Journal of Dental Research, 48*, 596.

Corah, N., Gale, E., & Illig, S. (1979). Psychological stress reduction during dental procedures. *Journal of Dental Research, 58*, 1347-1351.

Gale, E., & Ayer, W. (1969). Treatment of dental phobias. *Journal of the American Dental Association, 78*, 1304-1307.

Jerremalm, A., Jansson, L., & Ost, L. (1986). Individual response patterns and the effects of different behavioral methods in the treatment of dental phobia. *Behavior Research and Therapy, 24*, 587-596.

Kleinknecht, R., & Bernstein, D. (1979). Short term treatment of dental avoidance. *Journal of Behavior Therapy and Experimental Psychiatry, 10*, 311-315.

Kleinknecht, R., Klepac, R., & Alexander, L. (1973). Origins and characteristics of fear of dentistry. *Journal of the American Dental Association, 86*, 842-848.

Klepac, R. (1975). Successful treatment of avoidance of dentistry by desensitization or by increasing pain tolerance. *Journal of Behavior Therapy and Experimental Psychiatry, 6*, 307-310.

Moses, A., & Hollandsworth, J., (1985). Relative effectiveness of education alone versus stress innoculation training in the treatment of dental phobia. *Behavior Therapy, 16*, 531-537.

Mathews, A., & Rezin, V. (1977). Treatment of dental fears by imaginal flooding and rehearsal of coping behavior. *Behavior Research and Therapy, 15*, 321-328.

Miller, M., Murphy, P., & Miller, T. (1978). Comparison of electromyographic feedback and progressive relaxation training in treating circumscribed anxiety stress reactions. *Journal of Consulting and Clinical Psychology, 46*, 1291-1298.

Vrand, S., McNeil, D., & McGlynn, F., (1986). A structured interview for assessing dental fear. *Journal of Behavior Therapy and Experimental Psychiatry, 17*, 175-178.

See Also

Chapter 2. Anxiety - Stressful Medical Procedures
Chapter 29. Pain - Acute
Chapter 30. Pain - Chronic

14 Diabetes Mellitus

Assessment Strategies

Pinkerton, Hughes, and Wenrich (1982) define diabetes mellitusas as a chronic disease of metabolism characterized by an excess of glucose in the blood (hyperglycemia), usually by sugar in the urine (glycosuria), and frequently by the elevated fatty acid content in the blood. It thus represents a generalized disorder of the body's ability to adequately utilize not only carbohydrates, but proteins and fats as well. Symptoms may include abnormal thirst, hunger, increased urination, genital itching, and loss of weight and strength. [p. 299]

There are two major categories of diabetes: insulin dependent and non-insulin dependent.

Before attempting any behavioral assessment it is important to obtain consent from the patient's physician. The most important assessment information is the patient's blood glucose levels. These levels can be reliably obtained by the patient at home. Gross, Magalnick and Delcher (1985) describe using the AccuChek[1] test to obtain these levels:

> **To obtain a measurement using this method, a drop of capillary blood obtained by a finger stick is placed on a glucose oxidase reagent strip. After waiting 60 sec (signaled by the monitor) the drop of blood is wiped from the strip. The strip is inserted into the monitor. Following another 60 sec, a tone sounds signaling the operator to close the monitor test strip door. When this is performed the monitor electronically quantifies colorimetric changes on the reagent strip and presents an electronic readout of the individual's glucose levels in mg/dl of blood. [p. 502]**

These levels can be monitored twice daily: in the morning and late afternoon. Normal blood glucose levels are 80-120 mg/dl.

Fowler, Budzynski, and VandenBergh (1976) have developed a self-rated diabetic scale (see Table 14-1) that allows the patient to monitor typical symptoms associated with diabetes. Ratings can be made frequently throughout an assessment day.

For insulin-dependent diabetics, it is important to monitor the patient's compliance with the daily insulin dose. Other important areas to assess include obesity, diet, stress, and exercise. It may also be important to assess the possibility of an injection phobia.

Treatment Strategies

For non-insulin-dependent diabetics, treatment often focuses on the modification of weight and exercise. Hartwell, Kaplan, and Wallace (1986) found that a behavioral diet program was more effective than an exercise program in reducing the patient's weight and blood glucose levels. They describe the diet as follows.

---

[1] Available from Bio-Dynamics, Indianapolis, Indiana.

Table 14-1

SELF-RATED DIABETIC SCALE

Rating	Description
-4	Severe hypoglycemia Unconscious Convulsions Little or no recall of events Hospitalization
-3	Moderate hypoglycemia Some lapse in memory Insulin reaction requiring large amounts of glucose, etc. Strange behavior, i.e., acting drunk Nervousness, anxiety, and/or apprehension Confusion, difficulty in thinking Difficulty in focusing eyes Poor coordination Speech difficulties
-2	Mild hypoglycemia Hunger Sweating Cold, clammy hands Cold, shivering Tachycardia Able to recall all events Shaking Drowsy Weak
-1	Feel drop in blood sugar, but no insulin reaction Tired Hunger Mild weakness
0	Feel fine: No signs of hypo- or hyperglycemia
+1	Mild symptoms of hyperglycemia and/or acetone Weakness Thirsty Easily fatigued during mild exercise, e.g., walking
+2	Moderate symptoms Increasing nausea Weakness Starting to become dehydrated Headache
+3	Serious symptoms Extreme weakness Dehydrated Dizziness Blurred vision Drowsy, tired Difficulty in concentrating Severe nausea, and/or vomiting Kussmaul breathing Aches (muscular, joint) Difficulty in extending arms, legs, fingers
+4	Ketoacidosis requiring hospitalization

[Fowler et al., 1976, p. 108]

> **In the diet condition, subjects identified goals for the 10 week intervention and participated in goal-setting exercises. Participants monitored their eating behavior through the use of a diary and learned stimulus control by identifying external cues which lead to overeating or to the consumption of inappropriate foods. They were instructed in self-administration of positive reinforcement and modification of environmental cues for eating. Diaries were reviewed weekly and individual feedback was given to each subject. The role of cognitions in altering habits was described. [p. 451]**

Wing, Epstein, Nowalk, and Scott (1988) found no additional benefit in adding a self-regulation of blood glucose procedure to a weight control and self-monitoring of blood glucose treatment for non-insulin-dependent diabetics.

Relaxation training has also been found to be effective in reducing blood glucose levels in both insulin dependent diabetics (Lammers, Naliboff, & Straatmeyer, 1984) and non-insulin-dependent diabetics (Surwit & Feinglos, 1983). Lammers et al. (1984) used progressive muscle relaxation with twice daily home practice, while Surwit and Feinglos (1983) used progressive relaxation training combined with EMG biofeedback.

Learning to discriminate blood glucose levels has not been found to be an effective treatment for insulin-dependent diabetics (Gross et al., 1985).

Frontalis EMG biofeedback alone has been successful in treating one insulin dependent diabetic (Fowler et al., 1976) but produced negative results in another case study (Seebung & DeBoer, 1980). Seebung and DeBoer (1980) reported that the patient experienced daily hypoglycemia and severe headaches when attempting to lower her insulin dose after biofeedback treatment.

For More Information

Fisher, E., Delamater, A., Bertelson, A., & Kirkley, B. (1982). Psychological factors in diabetes and its treatment. *Journal of Clinical and Consulting Psychology, 52*, 993-1003.

This article reviews a number of diabetic problems to which psychological investigations are pertinent, including etiology, impact, adjustment, stress, adherence, and metabolic control. The paper discusses juvenile as well as adult related issues. The article can be obtained from E. B. Fisher, Jr., Department of Psychology, Washington University, St. Louis, MO 63130.

Wing, R., Epstein, L., Nowalk, M., & Lamparski, D. (1986). Behavioral self-regulation in the treatment of patients with diabetes mellitus. *Psychological Bulletin, 99*, 78-89.

This article reviews all of the behavioral treatment studies for insulin-dependent and non-insulin-dependent diabetes. Included are strategies to improve accuracy and compliance of self-monitoring, strategies for the modification of controlling responses, as well as for modification of stress, dieting, and exercising. Studies with children and adults are included. The article can be obtained from Rena Wing, Western Psychiatric Institute and Clinic, 3811 Oytara St., Pittsburgh, PA 15213.

References

Fowler, J., Budzynski, T., & VandenBergh, R., (1976). Effects of an EMG biofeedback relaxation program on the control of diabetes. *Biofeedback and Self-Regulation, 1*, 105-112.

Gross, A., Magalnick, L., & Delcher, H. (1985). Blood glucose discrimination training and metabolic control in insulin-dependent diabetics. *Behavior Research and Therapy, 23*, 507-511.

Hartwell, S., Kaplan, R., & Wallace, J. (1986). Comparison of behavioral interventions for control of Type II diabetes mellitus. *Behavior Therapy, 17*, 447-461.

Lammers, C., Naliboff, B., & Straatmeyer, A. (1984). The effects of progressive relaxation on stress and diabetic control. *Behavior Research and Therapy, 22*, 641-650.

Pinkeron, S., Hughes, H., & Wenrich, W. (1982). *Behavioral medicine: Clinical applications*. New York: John Wiley & Sons.

Surwitt, R., & Feinglos, M. (1983). The effects of relaxation on glucose tolerance in non-insulin dependent diabetes. *Diabetes Care, 6*, 176-179.

See Also

Chapter 2. Anxiety - Stressful Medical Procedures (regarding injection phobia)
Chapter 10. Compliance

15 Diarrhea

Assessment Strategies

One should rule out any underlying gastrointestinal pathology before beginning a behavioral assessment. Other common nonfunctional causes of diarrhea are an improper diet and the side effects of medication. A behavioral assessment should include a frequency count and a description of the antecedent situation. Each antecedent situation should be rated with a SUDS level.

Treatment Strategies

The use of systematic desensitization, to reduce the anxiety associated with situations that consistently precede diarrhea, has been found to be effective in treating diarrhea (Cohen & Reed, 1968; Hedberg, 1973). Additionally, a second hierarchy can focus on reducing anxiety related to the physical symptoms (e.g., abdominal pain or sweating).

Biofeedback (using an electronic stethoscope placed on the patient's abdomen), aimed at decreasing high peristaltic activity in the intestines, has also been successful (Furman, 1973).

For More Information

Cohen, S., & Reed, J. (1968). The treatment of nervous diarrhea and other conditioned autonomic disorders by desensitization. *British Journal of Psychiatry, 114*, 1275-1280.

This article describes the application of systematic desensitization to the treatment of diarrhea. There is also a discussion concerning the idea that diarrhea is a functional response to stress. The article can be obtained from John L. Reed, Senior Medical Officer, Department of Psychiatry, London Hospital, London, England.

Furman, S. (1973). Intestinal biofeedback in functional diarrhea: A preliminary report. *Journal of Behavior Therapy and Experimental Psychiatry, 4*, 317-321.

This article demonstrates the use of biofeedback in the treatment of five female patients with functional diarrhea. The article can be obtained from Seymour Furman, Psychiatric Center at Alvarado, 6310 Alvarado Court, San Diego, CA 92120.

References

Cohen, S., & Reed, J. (1968). The treatment of nervous diarrhea and other conditioned autonomic disorders by desensitization. *British Journal of Psychiatry, 114*, 275-1280.

Furman, S. (1973). Intestinal biofeedback in functional diarrhea: A preliminary report. *Journal of Behavior Therapy and Experimental Psychiatry, 4*, 317-321.

Hedberg, A. (1973). The treatment of chronic diarrhea by systematic desensitization: A case report. *Journal of Behavior Therapy and Experimental Psychiatry, 4*, 67-68.

See Also

Chapter 9. Colitis
Chapter 25. Irritable Bowel Syndrome

16 Dysmenorrhea

Assesment Strategies

Dysmenorrhea, or menstrual pain and discomfort, is primarily characterized by painful pelvic cramps. A gynecological exam should be completed to rule out any organic factors, such as endometriosis, which may account for the pain. Two types of dysmenorrhea, spasmodic and congestive, have been identified. Denney and Gerrard (1981) describe the difference between the two types as follows:

> **Spasmodic dysmenorrhea presents as acute spasms of pain, commonly experienced in the lower abdomen, radiating to the inner and frontal aspects of the thighs and occasionally to the lower back. The pain may be accompanied by diarrhea, nausea and vomiting. Symptoms appear on the first day of menses, often within hours of the onset of menstrual bleeding, and rarely last for more than 48 hours thereafter. Congestive dysmenorrhea, on the other hand, is seen as a variation of the premenstrual syndrome. It consists of dull, aching pains distributed in a more diffuse fashion throughout the body (e.g., headache, backache, breast pain, muscle stiffness). These pains are usually accompanied by other common premenstrual symptoms such as depression, lethargy, fatigue, irritability, tension, constipation, edema and weight gain. The symptoms of congestive dysmenorrhea appear several days before and are relieved by the onset of menstrual bleeding. [p. 309]**

A recent effort to validate this differentiation has failed to support distinct spasmodic and congestive categories (Nelson et al., 1984).

The Retrospective Symptom Scale (RSS) (Cox & Meyer, 1978) (see Table 16-1) can be used to measure the severity and frequency of the dysmenorrheic symptoms. For purposes of comparison, women who complain of menstrual distress have a mean score of 64 (S.D. = 48) on the RSS. The nondisturbed group mean is 13 (S.D. = 12).

Other behavioral measures include the number of invalid hours caused by the symptoms and the units of medication consumed. Daily ratings of pain and discomfort beginning on the first day of discomfort may also be helpful. In addition, a behavioral diary can help to identify any sources of tension both during menstruation and intermenstrually. The diary should contain ratings of general pain and discomfort, and cognitions that precede or coincide with the pain. The baseline diary should be kept for at least one full menstrual cycle.

Treatment Strategies

The most common finding in the assessment of dysmenorrhea is that anxiety is associated with the anticipation and the occurrence of the menstrual pain. Additionally, other stress-related situations often precede the occurrence of menstrual pain. Relaxation training and systematic desensitization have been found very effective for patients with spasmodic dysmenorrhea. The evidence of effectiveness with congestive dysmenorrhea is equivocal. Relaxation training alone, including home practice, may offer relief from cramping. Specific emphasis should be on uterine and abdominal muscle relaxation. Additionally, some

Table 16-1

RETROSPECTIVE SYMPTOM SCALE (RSS)

Name: ____

Date: ________

Please rate each of these conditions for frequency of and severity of occurrence, on the basis of your experiences of your last menstrual period. Total frequency refers to the total amount of time you experienced a condition during your last period, while average severity refers to the average level of pain or distress of the condition when it did occur.

<u>**Total Frequency Ratings**</u>	<u>**Average Severity Ratings**</u>
0. Did not occur	**0. Not noticeable**
1. Lasted less than 3hr	**1. Slightly bothersome**
2. Lasted 3-7hr	**2. Moderate bothersome**
3. Lasted an entire day	**3. Severely bothersome**
4. Lasted several days	**4. Very severely bothersome**

Condition	***Frequency Rating***	***Severity Rating***
cramps	________	________
nausea	________	________
vomiting	________	________
loss of appetite	________	________
headaches	________	________
backaches	________	________
leg aches	________	________
dizziness	________	________
weakness	________	________
diarrhea	________	________
facial blemishes	________	________
abdominal pain	________	________
flushing	________	________
sleeplessness	________	________
general aching	________	________
depression	________	________
irritability	________	________
nervousness	________	________

How much additional time did you spend in bed because of menstrual problems over the duration of your last period? Give estimated total numbers of hours: ___ hours.

Considering the number of pills (any kind) taken for menstrual relief and the number of days you take such medication, how many pills did you take last menstrual period? ____

[Cox & Meyer, 1978; p. 301]

patients will need to utilize cue-controlled relaxation techniques applied to a wide range of stress-producing situations.

Systematic desensitization can deal with the menstrual anxiety as well as with other experiences that produce anxiety and, therefore, affect the course of the disorder. Chesney and Tasto (1975) describe four excellent systematic desensitization scenes associated with the onset of menstruation:

1. **You are in your room studying, seated at your desk. You will go over your calendar and see that you are going to start your period this week. You also glance at all of the other things scheduled for this week—there is an examination in one of your classes, a paper due in another, and you had hoped on going to a few dorm activities and a few events at the Student Center. Because your period is coming, you wonder if you will feel uncomfortable this week and not be able to do all that you have planned. You are able to think about this, and to return to your studies remaining calm and comfortable.**
2. **You are in your room studying, seated at your desk. You glance at your calendar and see that you are going to start your period tomorrow. As you are sitting there, you are thinking of all the work you have to do tomorrow—and one of them is gym class. You wonder if you will have any pain and discomfort tomorrow when your period starts. You are able to continue thinking about this—remaining calm and comfortable, you return to your studies.**
3. **It is the first day of your period. You started this morning and are now hurrying across campus to your first class. You have four classes today and had planned to walk downtown to shop for clothes this afternoon. Now that you have started your period, you wonder if you will have any pain today, and if this pain will interfere with what you have to do. As you walk quickly to your class, you are able to continue thinking about the pain, but feeling calm you also think about the shopping you will do this afternoon.**
4. **You are sitting on the toilet and you notice that you have begun your period. As you are sitting there you are thinking of all the things you have to do today. You have four classes, and have planned to go on a long, quick walk with your friend. You wonder if you will have any pain and discomfort today. You are able to think about the discomfort, but remain calm and comfortable. [p. 248]**

An example of a scene related to the days preceding menstruation can be as simple as the patient imagining looking at the calendar and realizing it is ten days before her period. Both traditional hierarchies, and the non-hierarchal scenes described by Chesney and Tasto (1975) have been found to be successful. Goldfried's (1971) self-control modifications for systematic desensitization have been frequently used. Denney and Gerrard (1981) describe the procedure as follows: "While imagining scenes concerning menstruation, subjects were instructed to attend to bodily signs indicating menstrual discomfort or tension and to use these signs as cues to initiate the relaxation coping strategies" (p. 307). In vivo practice should follow the successful imaginary scenes. Both individual and group desensitization have been found successful. However, individual systematic desensitization assures that you can begin treatment during an asymptomatic period. Systematic desensitization has been successfully applied to dysmenorrhea by male and female therapists alike in 4 to 16 sessions.

Anxiety management training has also been found useful in treating dysmenorrhea (Quillen & Denney, 1982). Patients are treated in four two-hour individual sessions and are given a self-control rationale. Initially, the patient is taught relaxation training with tensing. Quillen and Denney (1982) describe the remaining sessions as follows:

> **During the second session, the subject was taught a briefer relaxation procedure eliminating the tensing exercises. She was also taught a technique for explicitly turning off sensations of pain and discomfort in the pelvic area by visualizing a warm, soothing liquid flowing from the abdominal region slowly downward to her knees, inducing a feeling of heaviness and relaxation in the muscles of her abdomen, lower back, pelvic area and thighs. The subject was told to press her hands on her abdomen to simulate the pressure associated with the onset of menstruation and then to concentrate on relaxing this area until the feelings of pressure were neutralized. This "turning off" technique was repeated for the pelvic area and thighs. The subject was supplied with another tape-recording of the briefer relaxation procedure and instructed to continue practicing relaxation each day until her next session. The third session began with the subject placing herself in a state of deep relaxation without assistance from the therapist. She was then asked to imagine a scene involving the beginning of menstrual discomfort and to become aware of the feelings of menstrual discomfort elicited by the scene. The subject then practiced turning off the discomfort using the relaxation-based procedure, signaling the therapist when the discomfort had been eliminated. Scenes were repeated three times, and five scenes involving different settings in which menstrual discomfort might occur (e.g., awakening at night alone in one's room, in class during a lecture, on a dinner date with a boyfriend) were introduced during the session. Homework consisted of daily practice in self-relaxation without the aid of audiotaped instructions. The fourth session included additional practice in relieving physical pressure in the abdomen, pelvic region, and thighs, as introduced during the second session, and relieving imaginally-elicited feelings of menstrual discomfort in conjunction with the five scenes introduced during the third session. The session concluded with explicit instructions concerning the application of the subject's self-control techniques beyond treatment, including prediction and early identification of dysmenorrheic symptoms and early application of relaxation to these symptoms. [p. 125]**

If the assessment reveals that the patient uses self-defeating cognitions that precipitate, or exacerbate, periods of stress or tension, then a cognitive restructuring approach is needed. This may be especially important for patients with congestive dysmenorrhea. At the beginning of any cognitive restructuring surrounding dysmenorrheic pain, it is important to ensure that the patient is well informed about menstruation and menstrual pain. Emphasis should be on the fact that dysmenorrhea can be self-regulated and controlled voluntarily.

Lamaze exercises have been found to be helpful in treating dysmenorrhea. Denney and Gerrard (1981) state that the procedure consists of:

> **(a) a simple explanation of the physiology of menstruation and menstrual cramps; (b) training involuntary muscle contraction and relaxation; (c) modification of pain perception by shifting attention to controlled breathing and visual fixations upon nonpainful stimuli; (d) tactile exercises consisting of light abdominal massage; and (e) physical exercises to increase circulation and muscle tone and to relieve pelvic congestion prior to menses. [p. 304]**

If the assessment reveals that the patient is being reinforced for her pain complaints, by receiving attention in her environment, an extinction program can be set up. Significant others can be taught to ignore the complaints and not reinforce the "sick" role. Additionally, attention and praise for improvement should be given.

Other adjunctive techniques that are common to pain management can also be applied, such as (1) directing the patient's focus of attention away from the pain and into other environmental cues; (2) using distracting stimuli, such as listening to music; and (3) using imagery that is incompatible with pain, such as relaxing in the warm sun in a quiet setting. Biofeedback generally has not been shown to be effective in the treatment of dysmenorrhea. However, one study (Heczey, 1980) used autogenic relaxation training combined with vaginal temperature feedback. This appears to be the most promising use of biofeedback with dysmenorrhea.

Amodei, Nelson, Jarrett, and Sigmon (1987) found that a coping skills package consisting of identifying and disputing irrational beliefs, the scheduling of pleasant events, problem solving and social skills training was not effective in treating patients with dysmenorrhea.

For More Information

Chesney, M., & Tasto, D. (1975). Effectiveness of behavior modification with spasmodic and congestive dysmenorrhea. *Behavior Research and Therapy, 13*, 245-253.

This study successfully used a brief systematic desensitization program to treat dysmenorrhea. The differential effectiveness on spasmodic and congestive dysmenorrhea is discussed. The article can be obtained from Donald L. Tasto, 701 Welch Road, Suite 213, Palo Alto, CA 94304.

Denney, D., & Gerrard, M. (1981). Behavioral treatments of primary dysmenorrhea: A review. *Behavior Research and Therapy, 19*, 303-312.

This article reviews four major treatment approaches: (1) hypnotherapy; (2) Lamaze exercises; (3) biofeedback, and (4) desensitization. There is also an excellent discussion of the definition and assessment of dysmenorrhea. The article can be obtained from Douglas R. Denney, Department of Psychology, University of Kansas, Lawrence, KS 66045.

Nicassio, P. (1980). Behavioral management of dysmenorrhea: An overview. In A. Dan, E. Graham, & C. Beecher (Eds.), *The menstrual cycle: A synthesis of interdisciplinary research, Vol. 1*, pp. 273-282). New York: Springer.

This chapter describes the psychological, affective and cognitive components of dysmenorrhea and presents a "mode-specific" treatment package. The book can be obtained from Springer Publishing Company, 200 Park Avenue South, New York, NY 10003.

References

Chesney, M., & Tasto, D. (1975). The effectiveness of behavior modification with spasmodic and congestive dysmenorrhea. *Behavior Research and Therapy, 13*, 245-253.

Cox, D., & Meyer, R. (1978). Behavioral treatment parameters with primary dysmenorrhea. *Journal of Behavioral Medicine, 1*, 297-310.

Denney, D., & Gerrard, M. (1981). Behavioral treatment of primary dysmenorrhea: A review. *Behavior Research and Therapy, 19*, 303-312.

Goldfried, M. (1971). Systematic desensitization as training in self-control. *Journal of Consulting and Clinical Psychology, 37*, 228-234.

Heczey, M. (1980). Effects of biofeedback and autogenic training on dysmenorrhea. In A. Dan, E. Graham, & C. Beecher (Eds.), *The menstrual cycle: A synthesis of interdisciplinary research, (Vol. 1)*. New York: Springer.

Nelson, R., Sigmon, S., Amodei, N., & Jarrett, R. (1984). The menstrual symptom questionnaire: The validity of the distinction between spasmodic and congestive dysmenorrhea. *Behavior Research and Therapy, 22*, 611-614.

Quillen, M., & Denney, D. (1982). Self-control of dysmenorrheic symptoms through pain management training. *Behavior Research and Experimental Psychiatry, 13*, 122-130.

See Also

Chapter 29. Pain-Acute
Chapter 30. Pain-Chronic

17 Fainting

Assessment Strategies

Fainting (vasovagal syncope) can be triggered by emotional factors. A medical evaluation is necessary to determine if the fainting is caused by cardiovascular or cerebral pathology. The behavioral assessment of fainting often includes a behavioral analysis of the fainting situations. Many patients experience the symptoms in response to a stressful medical procedure or at the sight of blood. Degree of blood phobia can be measured by the Mutilation Questionaire (Klorman, Weerts, Hastings, Melamed, & Lang, 1974). Alternatively, eight items on the Fear Survey Schedule (Wolpe & Lange, 1964) are related to blood phobias. The items are: open wounds, receiving injections, seeing other people injected, witnessing surgical operations, human blood, animal blood, medical odors, and the prospect of a surgical operation.

A behavioral test can also be used to assess blood phobia. Ost, Lindahl, Sterner and Jerremalm (1984) describe the following assessment procedure:

> **A 30 minute color videotape was shown... the tape was silent and consisted of four different thoracic operations containing large amounts of blood. The patient was instructed to watch the film for as long as she/he possibly could, without closing the eyes or looking away. They were also told that this was a very important part of the assessment, that they had to do their best, and that they could press a button to turn the film off should it be too uncomfortable for them. The behavioral measures obtained from this test were (1) the time (range 0-30 min) that the patient could watch the film; and (2) the experimenter's rating (0-4) of the patient's fainting behavior, where a 4 meant that the patient actually fainted and did not respond when talked to and 3 meant very close to fainting. [pp. 207-208]**

Heart rate and blood pressure measurements can be taken before and during the behavioral assessment. However, tachycardia often occurs prior to exposure to the phobic stimulus. Fainting is associated with lowered heart rate and blood pressure.

Treatment Strategies

Relaxation training can be successfully used to block the presyncope symptoms (McGrady, Guillermo, & Bernal, 1986). McGrady et al. (1986) used autogenic and progressive muscle relaxation combined with EMG and temperature biofeedback and suggest that relaxation can be successful in controlling fainting under the following four conditions:

> **(1) the symptom is conceptualized as a biphasic response;**
>
> **(2) enough behavioral analysis is done, perhaps with assistance from the significant other to delineate the "fight or flight" aspect of presyncope. In this case, increasing muscle tension was the crucial part of presyncope;**
>
> **(3) a sufficient number of sessions are provided so that the patient can induce the relaxation response quickly enough to block presyncope. The length of treatment**

> **required will depend on the patient's ability in acquiring the relaxation skills and the complexity of the psychosocial issues;**
>
> **(4) cognitive behavioral psychotherapy is offered to explore the role of fainting in the patient's life and to assist in formulating a healthier response. [p. 26]**

To use relaxation as a coping technique, it is suggested that the patient practice the relaxation sitting up or walking around, since lying down may slow down the heart rate and reduce the chances of the patient fainting. Relaxation can be combined with exposure to situations that elicit the fainting. Ost et al. (1984) describe a typical exposure program:

> **This treatment can be described as gradual practical training with components of prompting, social reinforcement and modeling applied in a flexible manner. However, the main part of the treatment consisted of: exposing the patient to slides of blood, wounds and injuries; watching a blood sample being drawn from another person, and from oneself; watching a blood-stained bandage; watching an operation; and visiting a blood bank and going through the routine procedure for potential blood donors. Each exposure session continued until the anxious and/or uncomfortable reactions had been, to a large extent, reduced or completely eliminated. During the first session the patient was given a rationale and description of the method. Then a specific analysis of the patient's phobic situations was made in order to arrive at suitable exposure situations. During Session 2 a hierarchy of situations which it was possible to use in the exposure treatment was made together with a detailed planning of the training. During Sessions 3-8 the actual exposure treatment was done and Session 9 was used for a review of the progress made so far, what situations remained, and how the patient could tackle these on his/her own. Finally, 1 session was reserved for extra training if this was considered necessary.**
>
> **The homework assignments consisted of continuous self-observation and recording of blood-phobic situations experienced or avoided. Furthermore, the patient had to expose herself to the situations worked through in the treatment sessions, at least once a week in his/her natural settings, and record the result of each exposure. [p. 209]**

Relaxation is contraindicated for use during the syncope episode because of the likely drop in blood pressure accompanying the relaxation response. Kozak and Montgomery (1981) found that using an exercise that emphasized tensing of the muscles at the first indication of fainting helped to prevent it. They describe a procedure in which the patient was instructed to use:

> **a skeletal muscle exercise which was expected to augment venous return and the rate of ventricular filling, and thus prevent the syncopal response. She was instructed to tense (and release) her skeletal muscles several times, employing three muscle groups (legs, arms, and torso muscles). Emphasis was given to tensing, with the client never instructed to allow her limbs to become completely limp, but rather to repeat short cycles of tension and release. [p. 318]**

Systematic desensitization has also been found to be useful in reducing anxiety to the stimuli that elicit the fainting. Babcock and Powell (1982) used aggressive or assertive responses to counteract the anxiety, and Cohn, Kron and Brady (1976) used angry thoughts to inhibit the anxiety.

Wardle and Jarvis (1981) successfully used cognitive strategies to treat fainting in one patient. They describe the techniques as follows:

> **Cognitive strategies were developed which involved the following components: (i) an intellectual and impersonal appraisal of the procedure, which was enhanced by showing [the patient] the records of each session after it was completed to provide a non-emotive account of a faint; (ii) statements about the safety of the procedure, an acceptance of completing it and the normality of some of the pre-faint symptoms. These were practiced for a few minutes before exposure, and during the first treatment session the therapist modelled and reinforced the expression of these and other coping statements. Three treatment sessions were given, followed by two generalization/test sessions. Sessions took about 1 hour and took place at two-week intervals. In one generalization session the venipuncture was performed in an impersonal fashion by a doctor that the patient did not know, and in the absence of the therapists. In the second the patient watched blood being taken from one of the therapists and then saw it dripped on her and on himself. Finally, the patient went alone to a pathology laboratory to have a blood test. [p. 16)]**

For More Information

McGrady, A., & Bernal, G. (1986). Relaxation based treatment of stress induced syncopy. *Journal of Behavior Therapy and Experimental Psychiatry, 17*, 23-27.

This article briefly reviews the behavioral studies done of fainting. It also presents a single case study where biofeedback is combined with relaxation training. The article can be obtained from Angele McGrady, Department of Physiology, Medical College of Ohio, 3000 Arlington Avenue, C.S. 10008, Toledo, OH 43699.

Ost, L., Lindhal, I., Sterner, U., & Gerrmalm, A. (1984). Exposure in vivo versus applied relaxation in the treatment of blood phobia. *Behavior Research and Therapy, 22*, 205-216.

This article initially reviews the previous behavioral studies on blood-injury phobias. A group study using exposure in vivo and applied relaxation techniques is presented. Included is an excellent description of both of these techniques. The article can be obtained from Lars-Goran Ost, Psychiatric Research Center, University of Uppsala, Ulleraker Hospital, S-750 17 Uppsala, Sweden.

References

Cohn, C., Kron, R., & Brady, J. (1976). A case of blood-illness-injury phobia treated behaviorally. *Journal of Nervous and Mental Disease, 162*, 65-68.

Klorman, R., Weerts, T., Hastings, J., Melamed, B., & Lang, P. (1974). Psychomatric description of some specific-fear questionnaires. *Behavior Therapy, 5*, 401-409.

Kozak, M., & Montgomery, G. (1981). Multimodal behavioral treatment of recurrent injury-scene-elicited fainting (vasodepressor syncopy). *Behavioural Psychotherapy, 9*, 316-321.

McGrady, A., & Bernal, G. (1986). Relaxation based treatment of stress induced syncopy. *Journal of Behavior Therapy and Experimental Psychiatry, 17*, 23-27.

Ost, L., Lindhal, I., Sterner, U., & Gerrmalm, A. (1984). Exposure in vivo versus applied relaxation in the treatment of blood phobia. *Behavior Research and Therapy, 22*, 205-216.

Wardle, J., & Jarvis, M. (1981). The paradoxical fear response to blood, injury, and illness—a treatment report. *Behavioural Psychotherapy, 9,* 13-24.

Wolpe, S., & Lang, P. (1964). A fear survey schedule for use in behavior therapy. *Behavior Research and Therapy, 2*, 27-30.

See Also

Chapter 20. Anxiety - Stressful Medical Procedures

18 Genital Herpes

Assessment Strategies

A complete medical examination is necessary for diagnosis and assessment of genital herpes. Drob, Bernard, Lifshutz, and Nierenberg (1986) employed the Client Posttherapy Questionnaire (CPQ), an expanded version of the Genital Herpes Questionnaire, to obtain information on the therapeutic needs of patients with herpes. Three major factors are assessed: depression, sexuality/pleasure, and stress/anxiety.

Treatment Strategies

A cognitive behavioral stress management intervention has been found to be helpful with herpes patients (Drob et al., 1986). The program combined relaxation training, rational-emotive therapy, and assertiveness training in teaching patients to cope with and control "life stress, especially those stresses associated with genital herpes" (Drob et al., 1986).

For More Information

Drob, S., Bernard, H., Lifshutz, H., & Nierenberg, A. (1986). Brief group psychotherapy for herpes patients: A preliminary study. *Behavior Therapy, 17*, 229-238.

This article describes a study in which a cognitive behavioral intervention was compared to dynamically oriented psychotherapy and to a self-help approach. A procedure for assessing the psychotherapeutic needs of the herpes patient is also included. The article can be obtained from Sanford Drob, Ph.D., Millhauser Laboratories, 3rd Floor, New York University Medical Center, 550 First Ave., New York, NY 10016.

19 Headache

Assessment Strategies

Migraine, or vascular headache, is characterized by a periodic, sharp, stabbing pain. The headache is often associated with nausea, vomiting, irritability, and may last from a few hours to several days. "Classical migraine" also involves visual, sensory, or motor prodromes and the head pain is unilateral. "Common migraine" is more likely to involve generalized head pain and is often associated with certain times of the week or the menstrual cycle. Cluster headaches is a type of vascular headache similar to migraines but occuring "in episodes that may last several weeks and are separated by 3 or more months . . . are of brief duration (less than two hours) and are present at least once every two days" (Blanchard & Andrasik, 1985).

Tension, or muscle contraction, headache can be acute or chronic. The acute tension headache is associated with a bilateral, band-like ache or tightness that usually lasts from 1 to 4 hours. Chronic tension headache is characterized by a dull, constant, bilateral, band-like pain that may last for a month.

Since approximately 10% of headaches have an organic basis, a physical and neurological exam should precede any behavioral assessment. Self-observation of headaches is the most frequently used assessment technique. The most important variables to observe are headache frequency, intensity, and duration. Intensity can be rated on a 0-to-5 scale as described by Blanchard et al. (1982):

> **0) no headache; 1) only aware of headache when attention devoted to it; 2) headache could be ignored at times; 3) headache painful but can continue to work; 4) very severe headache, difficult to concentrate: can do undemanding tasks; 5) intense, incapacitating headache. [p. 564]**

These variables can easily be recorded by the patient on 3" x 5" index cards with ratings for headache intensity on the vertical axis and time of day on the horizontal axis. An alternative to continuous recording is recording ratings hourly, every other hour, or four times per day (breakfast, lunch, dinner, and bedtime). An additional variable that may be important to record is the amount of medication usage. This baseline should be continued for a minimum of two weeks and may require up to four weeks to obtain a stable baseline of headache activity.

Summary information can be computed from the baseline data. The number of headache-free days per week tends to be a very important measure for the patient. The highest headache rating each week can indicate if the more severe headaches are being reduced with treatment. The headache index is the most frequently used summary score and is the average of the daily intensity times the duration scores. For example, if 24-hour continuous reporting is used, the headache index would be intensity times duration divided by 24. It is also possible to compute the index based on waking hours or other time sampled recording.

Blanchard and Andrasik (1985) have refined the headache questionnaire. Patients respond on a five-point scale ("never" to "always") to the following questions:

1. I awaken with the headache.

2. My headache ends within 24 hours.

3. I have sudden attacks of headaches.

4. My headache is worse at the end of the working day.

5. My headache is throbbing or pulsating.

6. My headache can be described as a feeling of tightness or external pressure on my head (bandlike or caplike).

7. My headache begins on one side.

8. My headache starts in the neck, shoulders, or back of the head.

9. My headache is associated with visual changes like seeing stars, blind spots, double vision and/or intolerance to light.

10. I have nausea and/or vomiting with my headache.

11. My headache gets worse if I strain, cough, or lift objects.

12. My headache is better if I can loosen up my neck muscles.

13. Aspirin, Anacin, Bufferin, Excedrin, Alka Seltzer, and similar drugs relieve my headache.

14. I have a prescribed medication to prevent a full blown attack of headache.

15. My headache starts during periods or relaxation.

16. My headache starts during periods of stress.

17. My headache is constant or nearly always present.

18. My headache is so bad I can't do anything when I have a headache.

19. During a headache the area around my temple(s) becomes swollen, tender, and painful.

20. My headache is present upon awakening but disappears __ minutes after I get up. [pp. 15-18]

It is also important to conduct a functional analysis of the headache behavior. The patient should be encouraged to keep a behavioral diary that includes the following information: when the headaches occur, under what conditions the headaches occur, headache-related cognitions, what increases or decreases the headache pain, and the consequences of the pain. It can also include the responses of other people, information on location, duration, and intensity of pain, as well as any medication use.

Some common antecedents of migraine headaches include certain dietary factors (e.g., fats, chocolates, fried foods, and oranges), changes in weather conditions, violent physical exercise, and sleep and hormonal changes.

Bakal and Kaganov (1976) have developed a "headache frequency record" (see Table 19-1) that combines frequency, duration, and intensity recordings with a brief functional analysis. Also included is a record of medication intake and a chart for localizing the headache pain.

The Coping with Headache Questionnaire (Holroyd & Andrasik, 1982) can be used to have patients rate their frequency of using various methods (e.g., medication, relaxation) to cope with headaches.

Many headache patients may also have significant depression. The use of the Beck Depression Inventory as a screening instrument is recommended. Patients who score higher than 8 on this inventory tend to do poorly with relaxation therapy intervention (Jacob, Turner, Szekely, & Eidelman, 1983).

Table 19-1 Headache Frequency Record

Code: ______________________________ Date: __________

TIME OF DAY		intensity						situation	activity	analgesic
		0	1	2	3	4	5			
A.M.	12									
	6									
	8									
	10									
	12									
	2									
	4									
	6									
	8									
	10									
P.M.	12									

(Bakal and Kagnov, 1976; p.124)

Treatment Strategies

Relaxation training should be the first intervention attempted for most migraine and tension headache patients due to the cost-effectiveness and reported successful results. Different types of relaxation training, for example, autogenic training, postural training (Poppen & Maurer, 1982), progressive muscle relaxation, and cue-controlled relaxation have been found effective. Some patients may need extra work on certain areas (e.g., neck and shoulders). The addition of peaceful imagery to relaxation procedures has only a minimal effect on treatment effectiveness (Phillips & Hunter, 1981).

Relaxation training can be done individually or in small groups and must include home practice. The in-office sessions can be audiotaped and the tapes given to the patient to use during home practice. At least one 20-to-30-minute home practice session per day is recommended. It may be helpful to review the patient's schedule in the home practice on a daily basis.

After patients have mastered the basics of relaxation training, they should be instructed to use the techniques when they feel the slightest indication of a headache. Significant effects have been found with as few as four sessions within a two week period. However, most programs continue for 6-to-8 weeks of treatment.

Janssen and Neutgers (1986) found autogenic training was superior to progressive muscle relaxation for patients with combined tension and migraine headaches.

Teders et al. (1984) found that a home-based relaxation program incorporating treatment manuals and tapes is as effective for tension headache patients as a clinic-based program.[1] This type of program involves only 2 1/2 hours of therapist time.

If the assessment reveals that stress or anxiety are precipitants of the patient's headache, then the addition of other behavioral techniques may be indicated. Individual or group cognitive techniques, including cognitive coping training and stress inoculation training, have been found to be effective for tension headache (e.g., Holroyd, Andrasik, & Westbrook, 1977). Patients should be given the rationale that changing thought patterns related to a stressor could possibly prevent the occurrence of a headache. The therapist can help the patient to develop competing self-statements that can be implemented at the first signs of a headache.

There is conflicting evidence as to the effectiveness of a combined cognitive and relaxation approach. Anderson, Lawrence, and Olson (1981) found that for some patients the combination of cognitive techniques with relaxation training may be more effective than either treatment alone. However, Holroyd and Andrasik (1978) found no advantage to adding relaxation training to a successful cognitive treatment intervention.

If the assessment reveals that situations related to nonassertiveness are antecedents to headaches, assertiveness training may be useful.

Systematic desensitization combined with assertive training has also been used successfully to treat the stress-related antecedents of migraine headache (Mitchell, 1971). These techniques combined are more effective in treating migraine headache than the individual components alone (Mitchell & Mitchell, 1971).

Other multi-component behavioral treatments have been used to successfully treat both tension and migraine headaches. For example, Mitchell and White (1976, 1977) used self-reporting, self-monitoring relaxation training, and 13 other self-control procedures (e.g., thought-stopping, habit reversal, assertion training, imaginal modeling) successfully in treating migraine and tension headaches.

If the assessment reveals that the patient is being reinforced for headache-related behavior, it is important to instruct significant others to ignore the complaints of pain and discomfort and reinforce "well" behaviors.

Biofeedback alone has been found to be effective for headache patients. Thermal biofeedback is generally used for migraine and mixed migraine and tension hadaches (Blanchard, Theobald, Williamson, Silver, & Brown, 1978). The thermal biofeedback is often combined with autogenic phrases, such as, my arms and hands are heavy and warm. EMG frontalis feedback is often used for tension headaches (Beaty & Haynes, 1979). These techniques may be especially useful for patients that do not benefit from the initial relaxation training (Blanchard et al., 1982).

Home-based programs combining biofeedback (by giving the patient a device to measure fingertip temperature)[2] and relaxation may be helpful for

[1] Copies of the manuals and audiotapes are available at cost from Dr. Edward Blanchard, Center for Stress and Anxiety Disorders, 107 Draper, SUNY, Albany, New York 12222.

[2] Available from the Conscious Living Foundation, Box 513T, Manhattan, KS 66502.

migraine headaches (Jurish et al., 1983). This home-based program included an average of 2.59 direct therapist contact hours (Jurish et al., 1983). Kohlenberg and Cahn (1981) have added cognitive restructuring instructions, assertive training, and time management techniques to the biofeedback and relaxation procedures in another home-based program.[3] Patients were only contacted by mail and phone. The combined treatment was effective for those patients that completed the program. However, there was a high dropout rate indicating many migraine patients may need some face-to-face contact in order to follow through with the home-based program.

Biofeedback, EMG followed by thermal, has been found to be somewhat successful in treating cluster headaches (Adler & Adler, 1976).

Relief from tension headache through the use of cognitive or relaxation training is generally maintained for 2 to 4 years (Blanchard, 1987). However, if EMG biofeedback was used alone, the benefits deteriorate over time (Blanchard, 1987). Additionally, there appears to be a progressive deterioration of effects for vascular headache patients treated with relaxation and thermal biofeedback (Blanchard, 1987).

Brief contacts (10-15 minutes, one time per month for six months) are as effective as additional booster sessions in maintaining improvement for both vascular and tension headache patients (Andrasik, Blanchard, Neff, & Rodichok, 1984).

For More Information

Adams, H., Feuerstein, M., & Fowler, J. (1980). Migraine headache: of parameters, etiology, and interventions. *Psychological Bulletin, 87*, 217-237.

This article defines migraine headaches and reviews prevalence and precipitating factors of migraine headaches. Behavioral interventions, including biofeedback, are also reviewed. The article can be obtained from Henry Adams, Department of Psychology, University of Georgia, Athens, GA 30602.

Blanchard, E., & Andrasik, F. (1984). *Management of chronic headaches, a psychological approach*. Elmsford, New York: Pergamon.

Included in this book are chapters on how to take a headache history, diagnosis, behavioral and traditional testing, relaxation, biofeedback and cognitive interventions, follow-up and maintenance. Other topics such as childhood and cluster headaches are discussed. The book can be obtained from Pergamon Press, Maxwell House, Fairview Park, Elmsford, NY 10523.

Blanchard, E., Andrasik, F., Evans, D., Neff, D., Appelbaum, K., & Rodichok, L. (1985). Behavioral treatment of 250 chronic headache patients: A clinical replication series. *Behavior Therapy, 16*, 308-327.

This article reviews the diagnostic procedures for migraine and muscle contraction headaches, describes assessment techniques, and provides a good description of the relaxation and biofeedback treatment protocols. Included is a

[3] *Self-Help Manual (Migraine Relief)* used in this study was published by Harper & Row in 1983.

discussion of predicting treatment outcome. The article can be obtained from Dr. Edward B. Blanchard, Center for Stress and Anxiety Disorders, 1535 Western Ave., SUNY-Albany, Albany, NY 12203.

Boudewyns, P., & Massey, E. (1982). Behavioral management of headache. In P. Boudewyns & F. Keefe (Eds.), *Behavioral medicine in general medical practice*. pp. 42-67. Menlo Park, CA: Addison-Wesley.

This chapter includes an excellent section on medical diagnosis and treatment and reviews the different types of headaches. Behavioral interventions, including stimulus control, relaxation training, biofeedback, and contingency management, are reviewed. The book can be obtained from Addison-Wesley Publishing Co., 1 Jacob Way, Reading, MA 01867.

Holroyd, K., & Andrasik, F. (1982). A cognitive-behavioral approach to recurrent tension and migraine headache. In P. Kendall (Ed.), *Advances in cognitive-behavioral research and therapy*, pp. 275-320. New York: Academic Press.

This chapter includes excellent sections on headache precipitance, vulnerability factors and behavioral treatment. Included is a detailed discussion of the cognitive-behavioral techniques. The book can be obtained from Academic Press, 111 Fifth Avenue, New York, NY 10083.

References

Adler, C., & Adler, S. (1976). *The pragmatic application of biofeedback to headaches: A five-year clinical follow-up*. Paper presented at the annual meeting of the Biofeedback Research Society, Colorado Springs, CO.

Anderson, N., Lawrence, S., & Olson, T. (1981). Within-subject analysis of autogenic training and cognitive coping training in the treatment of tension headache pain. *Journal of Behavior Therapy and Experimental Psychiatry, 12*, 219-223.

Andrasik, F., Blanchard, E., Neff, D., & Rodichok, L. (1984). Biofeedback and relaxation training for chronic headache: A controlled comparison of booster treatments and regular contacts for long-term maintenance. *Journal of Consulting and Clinical Psychology, 52*, 609-615.

Bakal, D., & Kaganov, J. (1976). A simple method for self-observation of headache frequency, intensity, and location. *Headache, 16*, 123-124.

Beaty, E., & Haynes, S. (1979). Behavior intervention with muscle-contraction headache: A review. *Psychosomatic Medicine, 41*, 165-180.

Blanchard, E. (1987). Long-term effects of behavioral treatment of chronic headache. *Behavior Therapy, 18*, 375-385.

Blanchard, E., & Andrasik, F. (1984). *Management of chronic headaches, a psychological approach*. Elmsford, NY: Pergamon.

Blanchard, E., Andrasik, F., Neff, D., Arena, J., Ahles, T., Jurish, S., Pallmeyer, T., Saunders, N., Teders, S., Barron, K., & Rodichok, L. (1982). Biofeedback and relaxation training with three kinds of headache: Treatment effects and their prediction. *Journal of Consulting and Clinical Psychology, 50*, 562-575.

Blanchard, E., Theobald, D., Williamson, D., Silver, V., & Brown, D. (1978). Temperature biofeedback in the treatment of migraine headaches. *Archives of General Psychiatry, 35*, 581-588.

Blanchard, E., Andrasik, F., Neff, D., Teders, S., Pallmeyer, T., Arena, J.,Jurish, S., Saunders, N., Ahles, T., & Rodichok, L. (1982). Sequential comparisons of relaxation training and biofeedback in the treatment of three kinds of chronic headache, or the machines may be necessary some of the time. *Behavior Research and Therapy, 20*,69-481.

Holroyd, K., & Andrasik, F. (1978). Coping and the self-control of chronic tension headache. *Journal of Consulting and Clinical Psychology, 46*, 1036-1045.

Holroyd, K., & Andrasik, F. (1982). Do the effects of cognitive therapy endure? A 2-year follow-up of tension headache sufferers treated with cognitive therapy or biofeedback. *Cognitive Therapy and Research, 6*, 325-334.

Holroyd, K., Andrasik, F., & Westbrook, T. (1977). Cognitive control of tension headache. *Cognitive Therapy and Research, 1*, 121-131.

Jacob, R., Turner, S., Szekely, B., & Eidelman, B. (1983). Predicting outcome of relaxation therapy in headaches: The role of "depression." *Behavior Therapy, 14*, 457-465.

Janssen, K., & Neutgers, J. (1986). Autogenic training and progressive relaxation in the treatment of three kinds of headache. *Behavior Research and Therapy, 24*, 199-208.

Jurish, S., Blanchard, E., Andrasik, F., Teders, S., Neff, D., & Arena, J. (1983). Home versus clinic based treatment of vascular headache. *Journal of Consulting and Clinical Psychology, 51*, 743-751.

Kohlenberg, R., & Cahn, T. (1981). Self-help treatment for migraine headches: A controlled outcome study. *Headache, 21*, 196-200.

Mitchell, K. (1971). A psychological approach to the treatment of migraine. *British Journal of Psychiatry, 119*, 533-534.

Mitchell, K., & Mitchell, E. (1971). Migraine: An exploratory treatment application of programmed behaviour therapy techniques. *Journal of Psychosomatic Research, 15*, 137-157.

Mitchell, K., & White, R. (1977). Behavioral self-management, an application to the problem of migraine headaches. *Behavior Therapy, 8*. 213-221.

Phillips, C., & Hunter, N. (1981). The treatment of tension headache—II. EMG "normality" and relaxation. *Behavior Research and Therapy, 19*, 499-507.

Poppen, R., & Maurer, J. (1982). Electromyographic analysis of relaxed postures. *Biofeedback and Self-Regulation, 7*, 491-498.

Teders, S., Blanchard, E., Andrasik, F., Jurish, S., Neff, D., & Arena, J. (1984). Relaxation training for tension headache: Comparative efficacy of cost-effectiveness with a minimal therapist contact versus a therapist-delivered procedure. *Behavior Therapy, 15*, 59-70.

See Also

Chapter 12. Conversion Disorders
Chapter 29. Pain - Acute
Chapter 30. Pain - Chronic

20 Hyperlipidemia

Assessment Strategies

Hyperlipidemia is an abnormal elevation in plasma cholesterol level (greater than 220 mg/dl) or triglyceride level (greater than 140 mg/dl), or both. Since hyperlipidemia can result from other diseases (e.g., hypothyroidism or poorly controlled diabetes mellitus) the patient should be evaluated by a physician prior to the initiation of any behavioral assessment. Laboratory tests are needed to determine a patient's plasma cholesterol and triglyceride levels. Patients should be asked to begin baseline reportings of the amount of cholesterol intake per day. Cholesterol levels in various foods are available in many popular calorie and food guides. Fetcher, Foster, Anderson, Grande, and Keys (1967) list the correct cholesterol content of more than 400 different foods. If the patient's cholesterol and triglyceride levels are elevated, it may be necessary to assess the following factors: exercise, obesity, smoking, and type A behavior pattern.

Treatment Strategies

The few behavioral studies aimed at reducing hyperlipidemia involve multiple target behaviors. Common to all approaches is diet modification generally aimed at reducing cholesterol intake to a maximum of 100 mg/day, and reducing dietary fat. Typical diets have been developed by Connor and Connor (1977) and Gotto, Scott, Foreyt, and Reeves (1975).

Behavioral treatment generally includes an educational component on nutrition. The use of a dietitian or nutritionist as a co-therapist may be needed. This educational component can include modeling of new behaviors followed by guided practice (e.g., a group dinner or shopping in a large supermarket). Weekly menu planning is usually included. Behavioral techniques that have been used to modify lipid levels in clients include: self-monitoring, stimulus control, and contingency management.

Foreyt, Scott, Mitchell, and Gotto (1979) describe the use of these techniques to reduce lipid levels as follows:

> **1. *Dietary self-recording* — Subjects were instructed to record all food and drink ingested, paying particular attention to foods high in saturated fat and cholesterol. They were also instructed to write down other relevant data regarding their dietary behavior, including times, places, and companions while eating. These food diaries were turned in to the dietitian at each class period who reviewed them in detail, writing down comments and suggestions for possible changes along with praise for appropriate eating behaviors. They were handed back to the subjects at the next class for their review.**
>
> **2. *Stimulus control* — Subjects were instructed in specific techniques to change antecedent stimuli eliciting inappropriate dietary behaviors. They were told to limit all at-home eating to one place, slow down the rate of eating by using a "Lay down utensils between bites" sign placed on the table next to their plate, and**

eliminate the effect the sight of food has on eating by storing problem foods out of sight. It was explained that good dietary habits maximize the chances of following a nutritious eating plan.

3. *Contingency management* — Subjects were awarded points at each class for attendance and completing behavioral homework assignments. Subjects with the most points in each class won two tickets to a play or ballgame. All subjects also completed the HELP Your Heart Pleasure Questionnaire, a brief form designed to identify various everyday pleasures, such as telephoning a friend long distance, sleeping late on Saturday morning, or relaxing in a bath. Subjects were instructed to reward themselves with these pleasures after completing specific behavioral assignments. [pp. 442-443]

Meyer, Nash, McAlister, Maccoby, and Farquhar (1980) also utilized the contingency management techniques that assigned points for success with eight out of ten dietary recommendations. Total points for all members of the group can be summed and posted on a graph in the room where the patients meet each week. These techniques are generally taught in groups and can be completed in two to three months.

Additional treatment for obesity, smoking, lack of exercise, or type A behavior patterns may be necessary if indicated by the assessment.

For More Information

Carmody, T., Fey, S., Pierce, V., Connor, W., & Matarazzo, J. (1982). Behavioral treatment of hyperlipidemia: Techniques, results, and future directions. *Journal of Behavioral Medicine, 5*, 91-116.

This review article describes hyperlipidemia and reviews the dietary, weight control, exercise, smoking, and type A behavior pattern treatments of hyperlipidemia. Included are discussions on preventing backsliding, the use of the family in treatment, and group support. The article can be obtained from Timothy Carmody, Department of Medical Physiology, Oregon Health Sciences University, Portland, OR 97201.

Foreyt, J., Scott, L., Mitchell, R., & Gotto, A. (1979). Plasma lipid changes in the normal population following behavioral treatment. *Journal of Consulting and Clinical Psychology, 47*, 440-452.

This article demonstrates the effective use of nutritional education and behavioral techniques to reduce lipid levels in people who are within the average range for the American population. The topics presented in the nutritional education are listed. The article can be obtained from John P. Foreyt, Diet Modification Clinic, 6535 Fannin, M.S. F700, Houston, TX 77030.

References

Connor, W., & Connor, S. (1977). Dietary treatment of hyperlipidemia. In B. Rifkind & R. Levy (Eds.), *Hyperlipidemia: Diagnosis and therapy.* New York: Grune and Stratton.

Fetcher, E., Foster, N., Anderson, J., Grande, F., & Keyes, A. (1967). Quantitative estimation of diets to control serum cholesterol. *The American Journal of Clinical Nutrition, 20*, 475-492.

Foreyt, J., Scott, L., Mitchell, R., & Gotto, A. (1979). Plasma lipid changes in the normal population following behavioral treatment. *Journal of Consulting and Clinical Psychology, 47*, 440-452.

Gotto, A., Scott, L., Foreyt, J., and Reeves, R. (1975). *HELP your heart eating plan* (booklet) (NIH grant no. HL17269). Houston: Diet Modification Section of the National Heart and Blood Vessel Research and Demonstration Center, College of Medicine - The Methodist Hospital, National Heart, Lung, and Blood Institute.

Meyer, A., Nash, J., McAlister, A., Maccoby, N., & Farquhar, J. (1980). Skills training in a cardiovascular health education campaign. *Journal of Consulting and Clinical Psychology, 48*, 129-142.

See Also

Chapter 39. Type A Behavior Pattern

21 Hypertension

Assessment Strategies

Essential, or primary, hypertension is a disorder of elevated blood pressure (BP) with no identifiable cause. Secondary hypertension, in contrast, is elevated blood pressure in response to an identifiable disorder. Hypertensives may be screened according to severity of the disorder by using the following classifications: mild (90 mm Hg—105 mm Hg diastolic); moderate (105 mm Hg—120 mm Hg diastolic); and severe (greater than 120 mm Hg diastolic) (Shapiro & Goldstein, 1982).

While the direct cause of essential hypertension is unknown, there are several etiological factors that have been identified. These include: family history of hypertension, diet and body weight, exercise and activity level, stress level, and smoking.

In assessing hypertension, a comprehensive medical evaluation should be conducted. Blood pressure may be obtained by the clinician or by the patient. A standard method of measuring blood pressure is described by Jacob, Fortmann, Kraemer, Farquhar, and Agras (1985) as follows:

> **At each visit, blood pressures were determined after five minutes rest, three times in the sitting position using the right arm. The average of the last two determinations was considered to be the blood pressure for the visit.... In order to eliminate adaptation effects... only the blood pressure data of the last three visits of the four visit measurement period were employed. Thus, the baseline blood pressure for a given patient was calculated by the mean of his or her blood pressure during the visits 2, 3, and 4. [pp. 36-37]**

Blood pressure levels for an individual vary over time and as a function of certain physical and environmental factors. Measurement conditions, therefore, should be standardized with respect to position of arm, body posture, persons present, and amount of time since last meal. Blood pressure should be taken at a predetermined time of day and after the patient has been sitting quietly for three to five minutes. Two to three blood pressure readings should be taken two times per day. The average of the readings can be used as the blood pressure level. In addition to measurement in the clinic, blood pressure level should be measured in the home by a family member.

Anxiety appears to be a mediating factor in many cases of essential hypertension. It is, therefore, important to consider an assessment for anxiety.

Treatment Strategies

Essential hypertension cannot be cured, but it can be successfully managed. Intervention should be immediate, as the patient is at risk for cardiovascular and renal disease.

Relaxation training has proven to be an effective intervention in the management of essential hypertension. Instructions for relaxation training may be given by the therapist or by audiotape. It appears that therapist-guided relaxation is more effective than taped instructions (Brauer, Horlick, Nelson, Farquhar, & Agras, 1979). Audiotapes of relaxation therapy have been widely used as an aid in home practice, but do not provide any added benefit to practicing the exercises without the tapes (Hoelscher, Lichstein, Fischer, & Hegarty, 1987). Brauer et al. (1979) instructed a group of hypertensive patients in deep muscle relaxation from a program developed by Marquis (1974). The intervention is described by Brauer et al. (1979) as follows:

> **During the first session, subjects were told that relaxation can help to reduce blood pressure by reducing muscle tension if used in a program of regular practice and application in daily life. The therapist then instructed the patient thoroughly in the technique which involved (a) assuming a comfortable position, (b) systematically and sequentially tensing and relaxing all major muscle groups in the body, (c) breathing deeply and slowly, thinking the word "relax" or "calm" during exhalation, and (d) imagine being in a peaceful, pleasant setting of their own choice. [p. 23]**

In addition, Brauer et al. (1979) gave relaxation tapes to these hypertensive patients for home practice and asked them to record their progress in relaxing. These techniques were effective in lowering blood pressure levels for these hypertensive patients. Brady (1973) developed a modification of deep-muscle relaxation called metronome-conditioned relaxation (MCR). He describes it as follows:

> **Training sessions in metronome-conditioned relaxation (MCR) consist of two parts. First, the patient is instructed to tense and then relax eight major muscle groups in a fixed order, much as is done in progressive relaxation training. . . . Then more general suggestions of physical and psychological relaxation are given while an auditory metronome is beating at 60 per minute. The instructions to "re-lax" and "let go" (the muscles of the body) are paced with the metronome's beats. [p. 729]**

Brady, Luborsky, and Kron (1974) applied MCR to hypertensive patients and reported success in reducing blood pressure levels. Glasgow, Gaarder, and Engel (1982) reported success in treating hypertension by use of progressive and meditative relaxation. They also incorporated generalization training by teaching the patients to use environmental cues to prompt use of relaxation.

There is no advantage to adding contingency contracting to the relaxation (Hoelscher, Lichstein, & Rosenthal, 1986). Exercise is an alternative intervention in the management of essential hypertension. Physical conditioning programs appear to be successful with populations of severely hypertensive patients (Reeves & Victor, 1982). Hanson and Nedde (1970) describe a conditioning program established for a group of hypertensive patients: "The group trained a minimum of three times per week for one hour. Muscle stretching and flexibility exercises, isometric-isotonic maneuvers, distance running, and competitive sports such as squash, paddle-ball and basketball were employed" (p. 49). Self-monitoring of blood pressure has proven to be an effective means of lowering blood pressure levels. Laughlin, Fisher, and Sherrard (1979) taught hypertensive patients how to measure blood pressure levels. Patients recorded three readings two times per day in their homes. Readings were usually taken before breakfast and after dinner. Self-monitoring resulted in a significant decrease in blood pressure.

Procedures may be combined in a treatment package in order to increase the effectiveness of the intervention. Ziesat (1977-78) included group interaction with peer reinforcement and competition, self-monitoring of blood pressure levels, and stimulus control to treat successfully a group of hypertensive patients. Family members may be included in the intervention. Wadden (1983) reported that spouse involvement in the patient's home practice of relaxation actually increased the patient's amount of home practice. Spouse involvement ranged from actively participating in relaxation therapy to providing the patient with reminders to practice relaxation.

Biofeedback has also been effective in the treatment of hypertension. Patients can be taught to lower systolic and diastolic pressure by attending to feedback signaling changes in blood pressure levels. Reeves and Victor (1982) describe the "constant-cuff" method developed by Shapiro, Tursky, Gershon, and Stern (1969) as follows:

> **In the constant-cuff method a standard cuff is placed around the upper arm and a crystal microphone is positioned under the distol end of the cuff over the brachial artery. The cuff is inflated and held constant at a pressure close to the subject's systolic blood pressure (or diastolic blood pressure). Following each heartbeat, if systolic blood pressure rises above cuff pressure, a sound is detected at the microphone. When blood pressure falls below the cuff pressure, then no sound will be detected following a heartbeat. In this way the system provides binary (yes-no) information about directional pressure changes relative to the cuff pressure on each successive heartbeat. After a trial of 30 to 60 consecutive heartbeats, the cuff is deflated for about 30 seconds and then inflated to a new level, depending on the main pressure on the previous trial. (p. 174)**

The effectiveness of biofeedback may be enhanced by the use of reinforcement. Benson, Shapiro, Tursky, and Schwartz (1971) describe the use of monetary rewards: "As a reward, after each presentation of tones and lights, a photographic slide, equivalent to $0.05, was shown for five seconds. The slides consisted of scenic pictures and reminders of the amount of money earned" (p. 741). Elder and Eustis (1975) used verbal reinforcement following reductions in diastolic blood pressure in a biofeedback type of treatment. If compliance with these procedures is a problem, you may need to utilize behavioral techniques for improving compliance.

For More Information

Glasgow, M., Gaarder, K., & Engel, B. (1982). Behavioral treatment of high blood pressure II. Acute and sustained effects of relaxation and systolic blood pressure biofeedback. *Psychosomatic Medicine, 44*, 155-170.

This article describes the results of a study of the effects of biofeedback and relaxation on the treatment of hypertension.The article can be obtained from Michael Glasgow, Ph.D., Gerontology Research Center, Baltimore City Hospital, Baltimore, MD 21224.

Jacob. R., Fortmann, S., Kraemer, H., Farquhar, J., & Agras, S. (1985). Combining behavioral treatments to reduce blood pressure. *Behavior Modification, 9*, 32-54.

A behavioral treatment consisting of relaxation training, restricted salt intake, and weight reduction is compared to the intervention of blood pressure monitoring. The article can be obtained from Rolf Jacob, University of Pittsburgh, Pittsburgh, PA 15260.

Laughlin, K. (1981). Enhancing the effectiveness of behavioral treatments of essential hypertension. *Physiolology and Behavior, 26*, 907-913.

This article describes assessment issues pertaining to the behavioral treatment of essential hypertension. The article can be obtained from Dr. Karen Laughlin, V.A. Hospital, Seattle, WA 98109.

Seer, P. (1979). Psychological control of essential hypertension: Review of the literature and methodological critique. *Psychological Bulletin, 89*, 1015-1043.

This article provides an excellent review of the behavioral treatment approaches to the management of essential hypertension. Included is the research on relaxation training, meditation techniques, and biofeedback. The article can be obtained from Peter Seer, Fachbereich Psychologie Rehabilitationszentrum, Sudring 15, 7812 Bad Krozingen, West Germany.

References

Benson, H., Shapiro, D., Tursky, B., & Schwartz, G. (1971). Decreased systolic blood pressure through operant conditioning techniques in patients with essential hypertension. *Science, 173*, 740-742.

Brady, J. (1973). Metronome-conditioned relaxation: A new behavioral procedure. *British Journal of Psychiatry, 122*, 729-730.

Brady, J., Luborsky, L., & Kron, R. (1974). Blood pressure reduction in patients with essential hypertension through metronome-conditioned relaxation: A preliminary report. *Behavior Therapy, 5*, 203-209.

Brauer, A., Horlick, L., Nelson, E., Farquhar, J., & Agras, S. (1979). Relaxation therapy for essential hypertension: A Veteran's Administration outpatient study. *Journal of Behavioral Medicine, 2*, 21-29.

Elder, S., & Eustis, N. (1975). Instrumental blood pressure conditioning in outpatient hypertensives. *Behavior Research and Therapy, 13*, 185-188.

Glasgow, M., Gaarder, K., & Engel, B. (1982). Behavioral treatment of high blood pressure II. Acute and sustained effects of relaxation and systolic blood pressure biofeedback. *Psychosomatic Medicine, 44*, 155-170.

Hanson, J., & Nedde, W. (1970). Preliminary observations on physical training for hypertensive males. *Circulation Research, 26-27* (Suppl. I).

Hoelscher, T., Lichstein, K., Fischer, S., & Hegarty, T. (1987). Relaxation treatment of hypertension: Do home relaxation tapes enhance treatment outcome? *Behavior Therapy, 18*, 33-37.

Hoelscher, T., Lichstein, K., & Rosenthal, T. (1986). Home relaxation practice in hypertension treatment: Objective assessment and compliance induction. *Journal of Consulting and Clinical Psychology, 54*, 217-221.

Jacob, R., Fortmann, S., Kraemer, H., Helena, C., Farquhar, J., & Agras, S. (1985). Combining behavioral treatments to reduce blood pressure. *Behavior Modification, 9,* 32-54.

Laughlin, K., Fisher, L., & Sherrard, D. (1979). Blood pressure reductions during self-recording of home blood pressure. *American Heart Journal, 98*, 629-634.

Marquis, J. (1974). *Relaxation tape and instruction manual.* Los Altos, CA: Self-Management Schools.

Reeves, J., & Victor, R. (1982). Behavioral strategies for treating hypertension. In P. Boudewyns & F. Keefe (Eds.), *Behavioral medicine in general medical practice.* Menlo Park, CA: Addison-Wesley.

Shapiro, D., & Goldstein, I. (1982). Biobehavioral perspectives on hypertension. *Journal of Consulting and Clinical Psychology, 50*, 841-858.

Shapiro, D., Tursky, B., Gershon, E., & Stern, M. (1969). Effects of feedback and reinforcement on the control of human systolic blood pressure. *Science, 163*, 588-590.

Wadden, T. (1983). Predicting treatment response to relaxation therapy for essential hypertension. *The Journal of Nervous and Mental Disease, 171*, 683-689.

Ziesat, H. (1977-78). Behavior modification in the treatment of hypertension. *International Journal of Psychiatry in Medicine, 8*, 257-265.

See Also

Chapter 10. Compliance

22 Hyperventilation

Assessment Strategies

Hyperventilation can be described as an "effortless heaving of the upper sternum and lack of costal expansion" (Masur, 1982, p. 100). Because hyperventilation can result from organic dysfunctions such as pain, severe febrile illness, mitral valve prolapse, and cardiac arhythmias it is important that the patient be assessed by a physician prior to any behavioral assessment. In some individuals allergies may lead to stuffed nasal passages, increased mouth breathing, and then hyperventilation. Cook (1979) describes the typical hyperventilator:

> **The person will sigh excessively and inhale more air than is necessary. A marked absence in the use of the diaphragm for breathing with a concomitant excess in the use of the thorax is also frequently noted. Excessive thoracic breathing can be detected by asking the subject to place one hand on the upper chest and another over the navel while breathing deeply. If substantial movement is detected in the upper chest in conjunction with an absence of movement over the navel, then it is likely that the subject's breathing requires correcting. [p. 32]**

Note the patient's rate of breathing. The rate of breathing is expected to be about 14 breaths per minute. Hyperventilation probably occurs when the rate of breathing exceeds 18 breaths per minute. However, some hyperventilators will not manifest rapid breathing.

Breathing observations can also be made in an environmental situation that the patient associates with the occurrence of the symptoms (e.g., shopping).

Hyperventilation can also be identified by instructing the patient to hyperventilate in the office. This is accomplished by having the patient take 30 deep breaths per minute for two to three minutes. Some clinicians have recommended as few as 20 breaths per minute, while others suggest up to 60 breaths per minute. Bonn, Readhead, and Timmons (1984) describe the procedure as follows:

> **The subject was asked to pant as vigorously as possible through both mouth and nose maintaining a rate of over 60 breaths per minute. It was explained that a predominantly upper-chest movement was necessary to maintain this rate, and the mode of breathing was demonstrated to the subject. The experimenter sat next to the subject, monitoring the rate, observing the degree of cooperation, and watching for the onset of distress. Although any suggestion of effects should preferably be avoided during the procedure, a minimal description of the possible effects ("slight dizziness and tingling") was thought to be necessary. . . . The subject was asked to signal the onset of any symptoms but was encouraged to continue overbreathing at the prescribed rate and depth. If the symptoms became distressing the procedure was stopped. With those patients who experienced severe symptoms a rebreathing bag was placed over the nose and mouth. [p. 666]**

The patient is observed and questioned to see if any of the typical symptoms occur. The patient can also be given a list of symptoms and asked to check the ones that occurred. The Hyperventilation Questionnaire (Franklin, 1985) lists the following symptoms: dizziness, breathlessness, tingling hands/feet, dry mouth, unsteady on feet, nausea, little stamina, trouble thinking clearly, trembling hands/legs, tight/pain in chest, seeing double, fear heart attack, depersonalization-derealization, headache, tetany, tingling face, breathing too much, cold hands, difficulty talking, feeling far away, crying, lump in throat, passing out, collapsing, blurred vision, panic, pounding, racing heart, nervous stomach, burning, tingling, crawling, rising agitation, feeling you want to run, muscular tension, feeling of wetting your pants, diarrhea, feeling hot or flushed, feeling you may die, feeling trapped/helpless, feeling the ground moving, exhaustion, feeling you are going mad, feeling you are losing control, feeling you may cause a scene. Patients can rate the degree of distress on a nine-point scale (0 = not at all disturbing, 8 = extremely disturbing). Patients who hyperventilate may also experience other symptoms that occur at times other than hyperventilation. Examples of these symptoms include: yawning, sighing, breath-holding, and coughing. Some of these symptoms may be more noticeable to others than to the patient.

Patients should be instructed to self-monitor breathing irregularities, sighing or gasping for air, for a one week period prior to treatment. Included in this assessment should be the antecedent behaviors and thoughts preceding these episodes. A general measure of anxiety (e.g., State-Trait Anxiety Inventory; Speilberger, Lushene, & Gersuch, 1970) may also be helpful.

Treatment Strategies

If the assessment reveals that anxiety-arousing situations precede the hyperventilation, then relaxation training or systematic desensitization may be needed. Some patients may need to be sensitized to the tachycardia associated with hyperventilation. This can easily be done by having the patient exercise to raise his or her heart rate. The patient should be instructed to take his or her pulse before, during, and after each series of exercises. The patients should experience the tachycardia without the negative side effects that they often experience with tachycardia.

Simple treatment to relieve the symptoms of hyperventilation after the patient starts to hyperventilate include breathing into a paper bag or having the patient hold his or her breath intentionally. Engaging in behaviors incompatible with hyperventilation, such as whistling, singing, or reading aloud slowly, may help to prevent the hyperventilation.

Many patients may only need to learn new breathing techniques. These techniques may also be needed for many of the patients whose hyperventilation is precipitated by anxiety. Lum (1977) suggests a three-part program. First, the patient should be educated about the effects of faulty breathing. Patients can be shown a list of somatic symptoms related to hyperventilation. Then the patient should learn to self-monitor breathing habits, and finally the patient should learn abdominal breathing. The self-monitoring of breathing irregularities used in the assessment should continue throughout treatment. Lum (1977) states that the patient "should be taught to develop a slower, more even rhythm of breathing with inspiration running smoothly into expiration followed by a pause before the next inspiration" (p. 10). Patients can practice diaphragmatic breathing exercises twice daily for 10-20 minutes. Fensterhein (1983) describes the diaphragmatic breathing exercises:

> **The patient assumes a slouched seated position—if the hyperventilation is moderate or severe I usually start in a supine position—with one hand on the upper chest and the other (or preferably a book) on the upper abdomen. The general instructions to the patient are to make the book go up and down as much as he/she can while keeping the upper hands completely motionless . . . . The therapist observes and coaches the patient until the breathing pattern is correct. [pp. 9-10]**

It is important to prevent abdominal tightening during expiration. It is also important to acquire a steady rhythm and slow rate of breathing, preferably 6-10 breaths per minute. Fensterheim (1983) suggests that the patient "make a 2-beat pause, saying to himself `pause, relax,' between the end of the exhalation and the beginning of the next inhalation" (p. 9). Cappo and Holmes (1984) found that inhaling quickly and exhaling slowly was effective in reducing physiological arousal. Practice can begin in a sitting position and progress to a standing position, walking in place, walking, and finally practicing during ordinary activity. Fensterheim (1983) describes how the training can be incorporated into everyday activities and then stressful activities:

> **The patient is instructed to take 2, 3 or 4 belly breaths at the correct rate, many times during the day. . . . The patient is instructed to do this every hour on the hour (regardless of what he is doing at the moment) and every hour on the half hour. He is also told to do it whenever he sighs, coughs, sniffs, or has a nervous laugh. The aim, of course, is to carry the patterns around during the basic training exercises into an overall and permanent change in the general breathing pattern . . . . In the stress counter exercises the patient is taught to recognize the first signs of his/her stress reaction or symptom exacerbation and to belly breathe until they markedly diminish or disappear. [pp. 10-11]**

Singh, Dawson, and Gregory (1980) have used aversive conditioning with aromatic ammonia to successfully reduce hyperventilation in a profoundly retarded individual.

For More Information

Clark, D., Sarkovskis, P., & Chalkley, A. (1985). Respiratory control as a treatment for panic attacks. *Journal of Behavior Therapy and Experimental Psychiatry, 16*, 23-30.

This article describes how hyperventilation may induce panic in many patients. A description of the treatment program, including voluntary hyperventilation, an explanation of how hyperventilation induces panic, and training in slow breathing, is described in detail. The article can be obtained from David M. Clark, Department of Psychiatry, University of Oxford, Warneford Hospital, Oxford OXD7JX, England.

Fensterheim, H. (1983, August). *Chronic hyperventilation: Office diagnosis and treatment.* Paper presented at the annual meeting of the American Psychological

Association, Anaheim, CA.

This paper describes the hyperventilation syndrome in detail and presents an extremely thorough diagnostic and treatment protocol. It can be obtained from H. Fensterheim, Cornell University Medical College, 151 East 37th st., New York, NY 10016.

Masur, F. (1982). A "realistic" behavioral approach to several common disorders. In P. Boudewyns & F. Keefe (Eds.), *Behavioral Medicine in General Medical Practice* (pp. 97-127). Menlo Park, CA: Addison-Wesley.

This chapter reviews the symptoms, pathophysiology and diagnosis of hyperventilation. The behavioral treatment strategies are discussed and a case study is presented. The book can be obtained from Addison-Wesley Publishing Co., 1 Jacob Way, Reading, MA 01867.

References

Bonn, J., Readhead, C., & Timmons, B. (1984). Enhanced adaptive behavioral response in agoraphobic patients pre-treated with breathing retraining. *The Lancet, 8404*, 665-669.

Cappo, B., & Holmes, D. (1984). The utility of prolonged respiratory exhalation for reducing physiological and psychological arousal in non-threatening and threatening situations. *Journal of Psychosomatic Research, 28*, 265-273.

Cook, D. (1979). Hyperventilation: Its treatment and relation to anxiety. *The Behavior Therapist, 2*, 32-33.

Fensterheim, H. (1983, August). Chronic hyperventilation: Office diagnosis and treatment. Paper presented at the annual meeting of the American Psychological Association, Anaheim, CA.

Franklin, J. (1985). *Agoraphobia: Its nature, development, maintenance, and treatment.* Unpublished doctoral dissertation, University of New South Wales, Sydney, Australia.

Lum, L. (1977). Breathing exercises in the treatment of hyperventilation and chronic anxiety states. *The Chest, Heart and Stroke Journal, 2*, 6-11.

Masur, F. (1982). A "realistic" behavioral approach to several common disorders. In P. Boudewyns & F. Keefe (Eds.), *Behavioral medicine in general medical practice* (pp. 97-127). Menlo Park, CA: Addison-Wesley.

Singh, N., Dawson, M., & Gregory, P. (1980). Suppression of chronic hyperventilation using response-contingent aromatic ammonia. *Behavior Therapy, 11*, 561-566.

23 Incontinence

Assessment Strategies

Incontinence of urine or feces, or both, necessitates a medical screening prior to any behavioral assessment. It is important to rule out any organic causes including urinary tract infections and diabetes. A more thorough urological examination may be needed if there are any difficulties in general urinary functions (e.g., painful urination and dribbling).

Choosing a behavioral assessment technique depends on whether the behavior occurs in the daytime, nighttime, or both, and whether the patient is able to keep records. For patients unable to accurately record their own behavior, an observer will be needed to complete the behavioral assessment. For nighttime incontinence, the sheets are examined. In addition, the patient is observed for the presence of wet or soiled spots. These observations can be as frequent as every half hour, or simply a single check before the patient awakens. Any independent trips to the toilet should also be recorded.

For daytime incontinence, hourly checks may be appropriate. Any accidents that occur between hourly checks should be recorded. To insure accuracy of recording, any wet or soiled pants should be changed immediately. For adults who are capable of keeping accurate records, baseline measures should include wetting incidence, the time of retiring, the size of the wet spot on the bed, and any spontaneous arousal during the night. The baseline should last a minimum of one week. Two to three weeks should be sufficient for most patients.

Treatment Strategies

Baseline recordings should be continued in order to monitor treatment progress. Out-patient, non-retarded adults with nocturnal enuresis have been treated successfully with a bell and pad conditioning device.[1] Turner and Taylor (1974) warn that these techniques may be difficult to apply to adults who are heavy sleepers and may not be awakened by the alarm. They also suggest that some patients may need an ear piece attachment so that others will not be disturbed by the alarm. The technique has not been successful when applied to geriatric residents in a nursing home (Collins & Plaska, 1975).

For hospitalized adult, non-retarded patients, an operant conditioning program can be attempted. Two of the successful programs have combined negative and positive reinforcement (Atthowe, 1972; Wagner & Paul, 1970). Wagner and Paul (1970) describe the set up of the ward sleeping area as follows:

> **The unit was arranged into three physically separated sleeping areas designated "nursery," "kindergarten" and "good section." Each area corresponded to the patient's demonstrated level of continence. The "nursery" was . . . as unpleasant a sleeping area as possible, e.g. sheets were changed only every three days in spite of**

---

[1] The enuresis alarms are available at Sears, Montgomery Ward, and J.C. Penny stores.

> **nighttime soiling, nothing was done to reduce the unpleasant odor, no cabinets, drapes, or rugs were available, and the oldest beds in the hospital were used. These patients were awakened three times each night and taken to the toilet. . . . In order to be promoted to the "kindergarten" area, a patient had to have seven consecutive days of daytime continence. The "kindergarten" area had . . . two beds with "bell-and-pad" sheets were placed in each cubicle. The sheets had the effect of awakening the patients at the first hint of nighttime soiling, at which point an aide made sure they went to the toilet. Generally the "kindergarten" represented a definite improvement in sleeping conditions.**
>
> **The "good section" had 10 individual rooms equipped with modern beds, a dresser, soft chair, a rug, and curtains. Adjoining these rooms was a reading room equipped with magazines, comfortable chairs, and a radio. In order to live in this section a patient had to be continent both day and night for seven consecutive days. [p. 31]**

Patients may also be rewarded with candy, cigarettes, access to meals, and praise. Rewards can also be given following appropriate use of the toilet.

A more simplified operant program utilizing habit training and a reward of wearing clean clothes, was found to be successful in controlling daytime incontinence with a diverse group of chronic psychiatric patients (Carpenter & Simon, 1960). Patients received a habit training program, which initially consisted of taking them to the toilet every two hours during the day until bedtime.

> **An effort was made to give these patients an explanation of the importance of proper toilet function. They were told that their cooperation in developing good habits might enable them to become more independent and bettter able to care for themselves. . . . The patients . . . were permitted to wear a clean suit of personal clothes as long as they had no accidents. All of these patients started the day with a clean suit of their own clothes, but if they became incontinent, they had to wear green fatigues for the remainder of the day. At the time of the change of clothing each patient was told the reason for the change. [p. 18]**

There is some evidence that a more simplified operant program may not work as well for geriatric patients (Monroe, 1963; Grosicki, 1968).

Chanfreau-Rona, Bellwood, and Wylie (1984) found that an operant reward program combined with environmental changes was helpful in treating geriatric patients. They made these environmental changes: "The three wards had the toilet doors and doors leading to the cubicles painted bright orange. A large picture of a lady using a toilet was stuck to the door leading to the toilet area. Plastic footsteps were stuck to the floors forming a line leading to the toilets" (p. 275).

A program of prompting, staff assistance, and contingent staff approval or corrective feedback has also been found to be effective in decreasing incontinence in geriatric patients (Burgio, Engel, McCormick, Hawkins, & Scheve, 1988). The intervention is described as follows:

> **Treatment consisted of regular staff provided toileting prompts (usually followed by staff-assisted toileting) and contingent staff approval or corrective feedback. . . . Staff approached the subject at the scheduled time and said, "(Subject's name), it's time to use the bathroom." If the subject did not respond, or if she agreed, she was taken to the bathroom. If the subject responded negatively, staff urged the subject to use the bathroom. If the subject continued to object, staff terminated the trial and returned at the next scheduled check/trial.**

If the subject did not object to toileting, she was taken to the bathroom where the pad and undergarments were checked. If the pad or undergarment was wet, corrective feedback was administered, e.g., "(Subject's name), your pad is wet. It's important that you try to hold it and let us know if you need assistance." Verbal praise was given for a dry pad. The subject was then assisted, if necessary, to the toilet. If she voided she was praised by the LPN. Finally, the subject was informed that staff would be back in 2 hours (depending on the initial schedule for prompting/toileting) and she was reminded to notify staff if assistance was needed in the interim. Also during this time, all occurrences of self-initiation and independence were praised copiously by staff.

If the subject's incontinence had not improved, or had improved but stalled after about 2 weeks, the delivery of prompts/toiletings increased to every 1 1/2 hours . . . and then every hour . . . for subjects who did not improve at the 1 1/2 hour schedule. The purpose of this procedure was to provide additional training opportunities for the subjects. If the subject improved at the more intensive schedule, the interval was then doubled (e.g., 1 hour to 2 hours; 1 1/2 hours to 3 hours). . . . If thinner scheduling resulted in increased wetness, a more intensive schedule was reintroduced. [pp. 349-350]

Nocturnal enuresis in the institutionalized retarded patient can be treated successfully with "dry bed" training developed by Azrin, Sneed, and Foxx (197). Table 23-1 summarizes this procedure.

Treatment is effective for most patients within the first three nights, but geriatric patients may take longer. Phibbs and Wells (1982) have successfully used the following program to treat a similar population:

To carry out the procedure, all nighttime staff are asked to:

1. **restrict all fluids for one hour before bedtime.**
2. **remind all residents to use the toilet before going to bed.**
3. **awaken the residents by speaking in low, calm voices and rubbing their backs.**
4. **guide the residents, if necessary, to the toilet.**
5. **praise the residents for compliance.**
6. **praise the residents for independent toilet trips.**
7. **ignore all accidents verbally, with no criticism. Residents were, however, awakened after accidents to have their sheets changed.**
8. **Give all residents with a "dry night" a gold star on their individual charts and praise them the following morning. . . . If any resident was continent for seven consecutive nights, the unit manager changed the waking time by making it 15 min. earlier during the pm hours and 15 min. later during the am hours. [p. 247]**

The time to awaken the resident can be determined by reviewing the baseline records for the most typical accident time closest to the resident's bedtime. This treatment takes from three to nine months to complete.

Azrin and Foxx (1971) have also developed a procedure for treating daytime incontinence in the institutionalized retarded population. Table 23-2 contains an outline of the procedures used.

The "pants alarm" consists of shorts that are moisture-sensitive; the shorts emit a signal if the resident urinates or defecates. It is important to have the resident remain in the toilet area, seated near the toilet, during the entire eight hour training session, except during lunchtime. The average length of training for

Table 23-1

DRY-BED PROCEDURE

- ***I. Intensive Training***
  - **A. Before bedtime**
    - **1. Bedwetter drinks fluids**
    - **2. Urine alarm placed on the bed**
    - **3. Potty-alert placed in toilet bowl [2]**
  - **B. Hourly awakenings**
    - **1. Minimal prompt given for awakening the resident**
    - **2. Resident instructed or guided to the toilet**
    - **3. Resident seated on toilet bowl**
      - **a. If urination does not occur within 5 minutes**
        - **(i) return resident to bed**
        - **(ii) at bedside give resident fluids and praise as reinforcers**
      - **b. If urination does occur within 5 min.**
        - **(i) give resident praise, snacks and fluids as reinforcers**
        - **(ii) return resident to bed**
    - **4. Praise resident for having dry bed (require resident to touch the dry sheets)**
    - **5. Resident returns to sleep**
  - **C. When accident occurs—45 min of cleanliness training and positive practice**
    - **1. Disconnect the sound of the urine-alarm**
    - **2. Awaken resident**
    - **3. Reprimand resident for wetting and direct him to the toilet to finish urination**
    - **4. Cleanliness Training**
      - **a. Bedwetter changes wet linen**
      - **b. Attendant reactivates urine-alarm**
    - **5. Positive Practice in toileting**
      - **a. Bedwetter lies down in bed for 3 minutes**
      - **b. Bedwetter awakened with minimal prompt after 3 minutes**
      - **c. Bedwetter directed to toilet**
      - **d. Repeat steps a, b, c about 9 times**
    - **6. Bedwetter returns to sleep when 45 minutes have elapsed since accident was detected**
- ***II. Monitored post-training phase***
  - **A. Initiation of monitored post-trainin**
    - **1. When resident has no more than 1 accident during a training night**
    - **2. When the resident correctly toilets on at least 50% of all opportunities during a training night**
  - **B. Procedure**
    - **1. Urine-alarm on bed**
    - **2. Whenever accident occurs, reprimand, cleanliness training, and positive practice follow for 45 minutes**
    - **3. No fluids, no hourly awakenings, no reinforcers**
  - **C. Termination of monitored post-training**
    - **1. Terminated 7 nights after last accident**
- ***III. Normal procedure***
  - **A. Initiated after resident goes 7 nights without accident**
  - **B. No urine-alarm, no reinforcers, no positive practice, etc.**
  - **C. Bed inspected each morning**
    - **1. If bed wet, resident remakes and cleans bed (cleanliness training)**
    - **2. If 2 accidents occur within a given week, the monitored phase is reinstated**

[Azrin et al., 1973; P. 430]

[2] The "potty alert" is used to detect urination in the toilet. It consists of a bowl that is inserted in the toilet. The device can be obtained from Leigh Valley Electronics, Box 125, Fayetteville, PA 18051.

Table 23-2

OUTLINE OF THE TOILET TRAINING PROCEDURE

I. When No Accidents Occur

1) Resident seated in chair when not seated on toilet bowl
2) Resident drinks fluids every half-hour
3) Scheduled toileting of resident every half-hour
4) Resident given edible and social reinforcer every 5 min while dry
5) Shaping of undressing and dressing during toileting
6) Resident given edible and social reinforcer following elimination in toilet bowl and returned to chair

II. When Accidents Occur

1) Trainer disconnects pants alarm
2) Trainer obtains resident's attention
3) Resident walks to laundry area to obtain fresh clothing
4) Resident undresses himself
5) Resident walks to nearby shower, receives shower, and dresses himself
6) Resident obtains mop or cloth and cleans soiled area on chair or floor
7) Resident handwashes soiled pants, wrings pants out, and hangs pants up to dry
8) Trainer removes resident's chair from use
9) 1-hour timeout procedures:
    - a) no edibles or social reinforcers every 5 min;
    - b) no fluids every 30 min;
    - c) chair not available;
    - d) continue 30-min scheduled toilet periods.

[Azrin & Foxx, 1971, p. 91]

profoundly retarded patients is four days. After completion of the training, residents are on a maintenance program. This program consists of six inspections, praise for remaining dry, cleanliness training for any accidents, delaying meals for one hour if the accident occurs prior to the meal, and omission of a snack if the accident occurs prior to snack time. One month after training, inspections can be reduced to mealtime and bedtime. If the resident is continent for one month, the inspections can be terminated. However, cleanliness training can be continued for any accidents.

Biofeedback of bladder pressure has also been found to be effective in treating incontinence (Cardozo, Abrams, Stanton, & Feneley, 1978).

For More Information

Azrin, N., & Foxx, R. (1971). A rapid method of toilet training the institutionalized retarded. *Journal of Applied Behavior Analysis, 4*, 89-99.

This article describes a comprehensive program for treating daytime incontinence in institutionalized retarded patients. There is a detailed description of the toilet training procedure and the maintenance program. The article can be obtained from Nathan Azrin, Psychology Department, Nova University, 3301 College Ave, Fort Lauderadale, FL 32314.

Azrin, N., Sneed, T., & Foxx, R. (1973). Dry bed: A rapid method of eliminating bed wetting (enuresis) of the retarded. *Behavior Research and Therapy, 11*, 427-434.

This article describes in detail the "dry bed" method of treating nocturnal enuresis in institutionalized retarded patients. The article can be obtained from Nathan Azrin at the above address.

Sorotzkin, B. (1984). Nocturnal enuresis: Current perspectives. *Clinical Psychology Review, 4*, 293-316.

This article reviews the definition and epidemiology of nocturnal enuresis. Treatment approaches reviewed include conditioning devices and dry bed training. Non-behavioral treatments are also discussed. Many of the studies reviewed focus on children. The article can be obtained from Ben Sorotzkin, 24 Tudor Terrace, Brooklyn, NY 11224.

References

Atthowe, J. (1972). Controlling nocturnal enuresis in severely disabled and chronic patients. *Behavior Therapy, 3*, 232-239.

Azrin, N., & Foxx, R. (1971). A rapid method of toilet training the institutionalized retarded. *Journal of Applied Behavior Analysis, 4*, 89-99.

Azrin, N., Sneed, T., & Foxx, R. (1973). Dry bed: A rapid method of eliminating bed wetting (enuresis) of the retarded. *Behavior Research and Therapy, 11*, 427-434.

Cardozo, L., Abrams, P., Stanton, S., & Feneley, R. (1978). Idiopathic bladder instability treated by biofeedback. *British Journal of Urology, 50*, 521-523.

Carpenter, H., & Simon, R. (1970). The effect of several methods of training on long-term, incontinent, behaviorally repressed hospitalized psychiatric patients. *Nursing Research, 9*, 17-22.

Chanfreau-Rona, D., Bellwood, S., & Wylie, B. (1984). Assessment of a behavioral programme to treat incontinent patients in psychogeriatric wards. *British Journal of Clinical Psychology, 23*, 273-279.

Collins, R., & Plaska, T. (1975). Mowrer's conditioning treatment for enuresis applied to geriatric residents of a nursing home. *Behavior Therapy, 6*, 632-638.

Gorsicki, J. (1968). Effect of operant conditioning on modification of incontinence in neuropsychiatric geriatric patients. *Nursing Research, 17*, 304-311.

Monroe, K. (1963). *Treatment of nocturnal enuresis among hospitalized neuropsychiatric patients*. Unpublished doctoral dissertation, West Lafayette, IN: Purdue University.

Phibbs, J., & Wells, M. (1982). The treatment of nocturnal enuresis in institutionalized retarded adults. *Journal of Behavior Therapy and Experimental Psychiatry, 1*, 29-38.

Turner, R., & Taylor, P. (1974). Conditioning treatment of nocturnal enuresis in adults: Preliminary findings. *Behavior Research and Therapy, 12*, 41-52.

Wagner, B., & Paul, G. (1970). Reduction of incontinence in chronic mental patients: A pilot project. *Journal of Behavior Therapy and Experimental Psychiatry, 1*, 29-38.

24 Insomnia

Assessment Strategies

Insomnia is a term used to describe disorders of difficulty in sleeping. Spielman (1986) describes the predominant insomnia complaints as "difficulty initiating and/or maintaining sleep, early morning awakenings, unrefreshing sleep, sleeping lightly, needing sleeping pills in order to sleep, and daytime consequences, such as fatigue and impaired concentration" (p. 18).

Prior to, or concurrent with, a behavioral assessment, a thorough physical exam should be conducted. The insomnia may be associated with a physical disorder, such as an allergy, or it may be linked to cardiac problems. An interview should be conducted with the patient to obtain information concerning the frequency and severity of the problem. History of drug usage should also be assessed.

The patient should keep a sleep record for at least seven days prior to any intervention. A sample sleep diary is shown in Figure 24-1. Additionally, a daily log of behaviors that may influence sleep should be maintained for seven days. A sample of this type of log is shown in Figure 24-2. An alternative method of record-keeping is the self-report Sleep Questionnaire (Lichstein & Fischer, 1985).

An additional source of information may be provided by the patient's bed partner. This report can be valuable as an accuracy check on the patient's report.

It is also important to determine the significance of the patient's sleep problem. Some commonly accepted guidelines for the definition of insomnia include: 1) an average of 30 minutes or longer to fall asleep (defined as early onset insomnia); 2) more than four awakenings totaling more than 30 minutes of wakefulness; or 3) less than an average of 6 1/2 hours of total sleep per night.

Treatment Strategies

During treatment, it is important to continue monitoring those areas of the sleep diary or daily log that are the targets of intervention. If the patient has erroneous beliefs about sleep, or sleep needs, he or she may need some basic education.

If during the assesment it is determined that prescription or nonprescription drugs are one possible cause of the insomnia, then it will be important to work out a program for withdrawal. Common drugs that affect sleep are caffeine, alcohol, sleeping pills, and tranquilizers. If a prescription substance is involved, the program for withdrawal should be undertaken in conjunction with a physician.

Two major approaches have been utilized successfully with insomnia: relaxation training and stimulus control. If the assessment reveals that the insomnia is stress linked, relaxation training is suggested. The premise is that if people can learn to be relaxed at bedtime, they will fall asleep faster. Many different types of relaxation training have been found to be successful in reducing latency to sleep (see review article by Lichstein & Fischer, 1985). Among the possibilities are: 1) progressive muscle relaxation, 2) autogenic training, 3)

Day	Tension in bed[1]	Minutes to fall asleep	Waking time	Hours Slept	Type of sleep[2]	Rest score[3]	Number of nocturnal awakenings	Number of times out of bed

[1] Rate on a 1-10 scale. "1" = Very relaxed, no tension; "10" = Extreme tension

[2] Rate on a 1-5 scale. "1" = Very sound; "5" = Very restless

[3] Rate on a 1-5 scale. "1" = Very refreshed; "5" = Exhausted

Figure 24-1
Sleep Diary

Day	Naps: Time & Length	Dinner time	Caffiene or alcohol (within 6 hrs. of bed)	Number of times felt drowsy during the day	Day fatigue* level	Number of times worried about poor sleep	Prebed activities	In bed activities

* Rate on a 1-5 scale. "1" = Well rested and energetic; "5" = Extremely tired

Figure 24-2
Sleep related behaviors

passive relaxation, 4) meditation, 5) self control relaxation, 6) metronome-conditional relaxation, 7) guided imagery, and 8) occular relaxation. Lichstein and Fischer (1985) describe occular relaxation as follows: "The technique involves six eye movements—up, down, right, left, around, and around the other way, each held for about 7 seconds and separated by 40 seconds of focusing on relaxing sensations in the eyes" (p. 337).

Systematic desensitization has also been successfully used with insomniacs (e.g., Borkovec, Steinmark, & Nau, 1973). The following scene was the only one used in the program: "Visualize yourself lying in bed . . . . Imagine your mind is racing and you're unable to fall asleep . . . . Imagine yourself turning your attention away from the disturbing thought and think only of relaxation" (p. 402). However, there does not appear to be any advantage in adding systematic desensitization to relaxation training (see review by Lichstein and Fischer, 1985).

If the assessment reveals that strong discriminative stimuli for sleep have not been established or discriminative stimuli for activities incompatible with sleep are present, or both, an operant approach utilizing stimulus control procedures can be used. The process involves teaching the insomniac to strengthen the association between sleeping and the bed, and to weaken the association between the bed and activities incompatible with sleep. The following program to achieve stimulus control has been suggested by Bootzen (1977):

1. **The patient should lie down intending to go to sleep only when sleepy.**
2. **The patient should not use the bed for anything but sleep. No reading, eating, watching TV or worrying in bed. The only exception is sexual activity.**
3. **If unable to fall asleep within approximately 10 minutes, the patient should go into another room and return to the bedroom only when the patient feels ready to fall asleep. It may be necessary to repeat this step if the patient then returns to bed and still cannot fall asleep within 10 minutes.**
4. **Have the patient set the alarm and get up at the same time each morning regardless of how much sleep the patient had that night. This step should also be followed on weekends.**
5. **The patient should not nap during the day.**

Additional stimulus control strategies have been suggested by Haynes, Price, and Simons (1975). They include:

1. **The patient should arrange differentiating stimuli situations for sex and sleeping. For example, soft music, dim lights or candles might be associated with sex.**
2. **The patient should not sleep in other parts of the house.**

According to Bootzin (1977), some improvement should be noted in two weeks; four weeks is a good test for the program. These techniques have been found useful in a wide range of patients, including older adults (Puder, Lacks, Bartelson, & Storandt, 1983) and patients with sleep-maintenance insomnia (Morin & Azrin, 1987).

Cassette programs for the patient are available. However, Haynes et al. (1974) found that therapist contact had a small but significant effect on sleep behaviors in insomniacs. The results of this study suggested that even if a patient is assigned a home cassette program, weekly contact with the therapist would add to the overall effectiveness of the program.

Stimulus control procedures tend to produce the greatest reduction in latency to sleep (Lichstein & Fischer, 1985).

The simple use of sleep habits and practices conducive to good sleep is called sleep hygiene. These practices include:

> **(a) no alcohol within four hours of bedtime, (b) no caffeine after 4 p.m., (c) no vigorous exercise within two hours of bedtime, (d) no napping during the day, (e) engaging in nonspecific relaxing behaviors before bedtime, (f) not going to bed hungry or thirsty, and (g) sleeping in a comfortable environment, including regulation of noise, temperature, and mattress quality. [Scholcket, Bertelson, & Lacks, p. 186]**

Many stimulus control programs for insomnia often include sleep hygiene. Sleep hygiene alone has been found to be as effective as stimulus control or meditation for sleep maintenance insomnia (Scholcket et al., 1988). However, after a six-week followup, the patients rated the sleep hygiene treatment less favorably and were more likely to still consider themselves insomniacs than the patients in the stimulus control or meditation treatments (Scholcket et al., 1988).

If the assessment indicates that a cognitive component, such as racing thoughts, contributes to the insomnia, then the use of thought stopping may be appropriate. These thoughts can then be replaced by positive self-instructions. Rational restructuring may also be a useful adjunctive treatment (Thoresen, Coates, Kirmil-Gray, & Rosekind, 1981).

An additional intervention that has been used successfully with insomniacs is paradoxical intention. Ascher and Turner (1980) describe the procedure as follows:

> **. . . clients were fully informed of therapist's reasons for employing this procedure with insomnia. Clients were instructed to remain awake for as long as was possible under conditions natural for the onset and maintenance of sleep, i.e. lights out, clients lying in bed, quiet surroundings, etc. Clients were cautioned not to move around or engage in behavior specifically designed to prevent sleep. [p. 123]**

Ascher and Turner (1980) also found that explaining the therapeutic rationale truthfully to the patient was more effective than deceiving the patient. Lacks, Bertelson, Gans, and Kunkel (1983) found that stimulus control techniques were superior to relaxation training and paradoxical intention for treating sleep-onset insomnia of any severity. However, Ladouceur and Gros-Louis (1986) found no difference between paradoxical intention and stimulus control techniques.

Stam and Bultz (1986) successfully employed a combination of somatic focusing and imagery training in the treatment of a patient with insomnia secondary to cancer and chemotherapy. The intervention is described as follows:

> **The somatic focusing consisted of progressive muscle relaxation training (Bernstein & Borkovec, 1973) with the omission of instructions to alternately tense and relax the various muscle groups. The client was asked to focus on feelings of tension in 16 major muscle groups and to release that tension without first tightening the muscles. Instead, he was asked to relax the muscle, imagine it becoming limp and**

> **heavy and allow feelings of relaxation to replace the tension. Each session was begun with the somatic focusing exercise.**
>
> **The imagery training component of the treatment consisted of instructions to focus attention on images with the eyes closed. Pictures of a series of common objects were presented as prompts (a book, a candle, a clock, a cup and a bowl) and were faded after the client reported being able to visualize them. . . . The client was instructed to concentrate on the specific features, color and movement of the images. He visualized each object for 2-3 min while following guided imagery instructions that were also gradually faded. Both somatic focusing and imagery training were to be practiced at home daily. [pp. 34-35]**

Frontalis EMG biofeedback has generally been found to be effective for insomnia (e.g., Nicassio, Boylan, & McCabe, 1982; VanderPlate & Eno, 1983).

For More Information

Bootzin, R. (1977). *Behavioral treatment of insomnia: A clinician's guide and self-management techniques for controlling insomnia (*Audiocassette). New York: BMA Audiocassette Programs

Two tapes are included: one for the clinician and one for the patient. Behavioral assessment and treatment are covered. Also included is a manual containing assessment aids and other relevant references. The tapes can be obtained from BMA Audiocassette Programs, 200 Park Ave. South, New York, NY 10003.

Lacks, P. (1987). *Behavioral treatment for persistent insomnia.* New York: Pergamon.

This practical handbook includes a discussion of the theories of insomnia, diagnosis, and treatment. A four-week stimulus control program is included. The book can be obtained from Pergamon Press, Fairview Park, Elmsford, NY 10523.

Lichstein, K., & Fischer, S. (1985). Insomnia. In M. Hersen & A. Bellack (Eds.), *Handbook of clinical behavior therapy* (pp. 319-352). New York: Plenum.

This chapter defines the various categories of insomnia and provides a thorough review of assessment strategies and treatments, including medical and psychological. Included is an excellent evaluation of the behavior therapy studies and a case study illustration. The book can be obtained from Plenum Press, 233 Spring St., New York, NY 10013.

Spielman, A. (1986). Assessment of insomnia. *Clinical Psychology Review, 6,* 11-25.

This article thoroughly reviews all of the insomnia diagnoses. A detailed discussion of taking a sleep history is included. The article can be obtained from Arthur J. Spielman, Ph.D., Department of Psychology, City College of New York, Convent Ave. and 138th St., New York, NY 10031.

References

Ascher, L., & Turner, R. (1980). A comparison of two methods for the administration of paradoxical intention. *Behavior Research and Therapy, 18,* 121-126.

Bootzin, R. (1977). *Behavioral treatment of insomnia: A clinician's guide and self-management techniques for controlling insomnia.* New York: Audiocassette Programs.

Borkovec, T., Steinmark, S., & Nau, S. (1973). Relaxation training and single-item desensitization in the group treatment of insomnia. *Journal of Behavior Therapy and Experimental Psychiatry, 4,* 401-404.

Haynes, S., Price, G., & Simons, J. (1975). Stimulus control treatment of insomnia. *Journal of Behavior Therapy and Experimental Psychiatry, 6,* 279-282.

Lacks, P., Bertelson, A., Gans, L., & Kunkel, J. (1983). The effectiveness of three behavioral treatments for different degrees of sleep onset insomnia. *Behavior Therapy, 14,* 593-605.

Ladouceur, R., & Gros-Louis, Y. (1986). Paradoxical intervention vs stimulus control in the treatment of insomnia. *Journal of Behavior Therapy and Experimental Psychiatry, 17,* 267-269.

Lichstein, K., & Fischer, S. (1985). Insomnia. In M. Hersen & A. Bellack (Eds.), *Handbook of clinical behavior therapy* (pp. 319-352). New York: Plenum.

Morin, C., & Azpin, N. (1987). Stimulus controlled imagery training in treating sleep-maintenance insomnia. *Journal of Consulting and Clinical Psychology, 55,* 260-262.

Nicassio, P., Boylan, M., & McCabe, T. (1982). Progressive relaxation, EMG biofeedback and biofeedback placebo in the treatment of sleep-onset insomnia. *British Journal of Medical Psychology, 55,* 159-166.

Puder, R., Lacks, P., Bertelson, A., & Storandt, M. (1983). Short-term stimulus control treatment of insomnia in older adults. *Journal of Behavior Therapy and Experimental Psychiatry, 14,* 424-429.

Scholcket, S., Bertelson, A., & Lacks, P. (1988). Is sleep hygiene a sufficient treatment for sleep-maintenance insomnia? *Behavior Therapy, 19,* 183-190.

Spielman, A. (1986). Assessment of insomnia. *Clinical Psychology Review, 6,* 11-25.

Stam, H., & Bultz, B. (1986). The treatment of severe insomnia in a cancer patient. *Journal of Behavior Therapy and Experimental Psychiatry, 7,* 33-37.

Thoresen, C., Coates, T., Kirmil-Gray, K., & Rosekind, M. (1981). Behavioral self-management in treating sleep-maintenance insomnia. *Journal of Behavioral Medicine, 4,* 41-52.

VanderPlate, C., & Eno, E. (1983). Electromyograph biofeedback and sleep onset insomnia: Comparison of treatment and placebo. *Behavioral Engineering, 8*, 146-153.

25 Irritable Bowel Syndrome

Assessment Strategies

Irritable bowel syndrome (IBS) is characterized by abdominal pain and either constipation or diarrhea in the absence of any anatomical cause. A behavioral assessment should include a daily record of the patient's major gastrointestinal symptoms. Typical categories include: medication usage, ratings of pain and tenderness, discomfort, restriction of activity, fatigue, flatulence, belching, nausea, and the number of normal and abnormal bowel movements. Additionally, a behavioral diary consisting of the antecedents and consequences of abdominal pain, constipation, or diarrhea may be helpful. The patient's relatives can also be asked to keep a record of the frequency of the patient's verbal complaints of pain, constipation, or diarrhea. A general measure of anxiety (e.g., the State-Trait Anxiety Inventory) may also be helpful.

Treatment Strategies

The major interventions used for IBS fall into the general category of stress management techniques. The behavioral diary can be used to identify stress-related situations in the patient's life. Bennett and Wilkinson (1985) used an eight-week program of relaxation training and cognitive self-instructional training to successfully treat 12 patients with IBS. Patients were also educated about bowel functions at the start of the program. Neff and Blanchard (1987) combined relaxation training, thermal biofeedback, cognitive coping strategies, and the provision of educational information in sucessfully treating IBS patients. They describe the program as follows:

> During therapy, participants were taught to reduce gradually the number of muscle groups used, from sixteen to four. Concurrently, participants were taught to relax by recalling sensations of relaxation or release they felt when they practiced using tension-release cycles. A cassette tape of the initial relaxation session was offered to all participants.
>
> Participants were instructed to take slow, deep, diaphragmatic breaths to help them relax quickly in everyday situations. Participants were encouraged to practice the exercises at least once a day and were asked to record the depth of relaxation achieved.
>
> *Thermal biofeedback treatment.* After relaxation therapy, participants were given five sessions of thermal biofeedback treatment. This self-contol strategy was designed to help participants achieve an even deeper relaxation by allowing the autonomic response of vasodilation of the blood vessels in the hand to occur. . . . Participants were provided with a small thermometer to allow them to practice at home.
>
> *Training in stress-coping strategies.* A final aspect of treatment involved the implementation of stress-coping strategies. This was intended to help participants first become more aware of their perceptions of and responses to stressful situ-

ations, and then learn more effective strategies for dealing with these situations. Throughout treatment, participants were asked to become more aware of muscle tension while learning ways to reduce stress.

These coping strategies were intended to help participants deal more effectively with stressful situations by actively identifying situations that contribute to their symptoms. These strategies should then enable participants to reduce stress, by avoiding these situations or developing more effective ways to cope with them. [pp. 73-74]

For More Information

Bennett, P., & Wilkinson, S. (1985). A comparison of psychological and medical treatment of the irritable bowel syndrome. *British Journal of Clinical Psychology, 24*, 215-216.

This study compares a stress management package to drug intervention in treating a group of IBS patients. The article can be obtained from Paul Bennett, Department of Psychology, Whitchurch Hospital, Cardiff, CF47XD, England.

Blanchard, E., Schwartz, S., & Radnitz, C. (1987). Psychological assessment and treatment of irritable bowel syndrome. *Behavior Modification, 11*, 348-372.

This article initially defines the syndrome, discusses the epidemiology and medical treatment. Psychological assessment and treatment are reviewed, including behavioral and non-behavioral studies. Recent behavioral studies utilizing relaxation, thermal biofeedback, and cognitive stress-coping techniques are also discussed. The article can be obtained from Dr. Edward Blanchard, Center for Stress and Anxiety Disorders, 1535 Western Ave., SUNY-Albany, Albany, NY 12203.

References

Bennett, P., & Wilkinson, S. (1985). A comparison of psychological and medical treatment of the irritable bowel syndrome. *British Journal of Clinical Psychology, 24*, 215-216.

Neff, D., & Blanchard, E. (1987). A multi-component treatment for irritable bowel syndrome. *Behavior Therapy, 18*, 70-83.

See Also

Chapter 10. Constipation
Chapter 15. Diarrhea
Chapter 30. Pain - Chronic

26 Menopausal Hot Flashes

Assessment Strategies

Hot flash is the term used to describe a phenomenon that occurs in a significant proportion of menopausal women. Stevenson and Delprato (1983) describe the hot flash as "a sudden hot feeling accompanied by flushing of the face and sometimes sweating" (p. 137).

Assessment should include a complete physical evaluation and clinical interview. Prior to intervention, the clinician should obtain a baseline measure of frequency and duration of hot flashes. Germaine and Freedman (1984) employed an objective measure, the Heat Stress Test (HST), to elicit the hot flash. They describe the procedure as follows:

> **HST 1 began with a 10-min baseline period followed by the application of the heat stressor (two circulation water pads maintained at $42^{oC} \pm 1^{oC)}$ to the subject's torso while supine on a bed in a 23^{oC} temperature and humidity controlled room. Subjects wore only a light cotton gown. A woolen blanket was loosely draped over the subject, whose arms and hands rested by her side and above the blanket throughout the test, which lasted 20 min. Subjects were instructed to signal the earliest perception of a hot flash by pushing a hand-held button. [p. 1073]**

In addition to the HST, Germaine and Freedman (1984) also provided patients with a symptom diary in which they were instructed to record the occurrence of each hot flash.

Treatment Strategies

Relaxation training has been used successfully in reducing the frequency of menopausal hot flashes. Germaine and Freedman (1984) first gave women information about the physiology of the hot flash and relaxation. Relaxation was presented as a method of controlling the physiologic arousal of the hot flash. Patients received six sessions of standard muscle relaxation and were instructed to practice the relaxation twice daily.

Stevenson and Delprato (1983) developed a multicomponent program to treat a group of menopausal women. This program included relaxation training, self-control techniques, contingency contracting, and temperature feedback.

> **The training period took place over 12 weeks, during which 10 sessions were held. At the first session, the therapist administered relaxation instructions . . . and gave P a tape recording for home practice; relaxation training continued in session 2. For sessions 3 and 4, the therapist used each P's hot flash records to construct individualized hierarchies of life situations in which Ps reported flashes. Each was given her hierarchy and instructed first to imagine the lowest situation (minimally problematic). She was instructed to use relaxation to counteract the hot flash or**

> **tension as soon as either was detected in response to imagining the situation. Once P quickly attenuated flashing and/or tension with the lowest hierarchical situation, she began the same process with the next higher situation and progressed up the hierarchy. The hierarchy was taken home for practice.**
>
> **Thought stopping and semantic counterconditioning . . . were introduced in session 5. Ps were taught to identify self-thoughts that were compatible with flashes and tension, to stop them, and to replace them with self-statements that were relaxing and non-stressing. The use of cool thoughts and images . . . as a coping skill for hot flashes and marital contingency contracting . . . for reducing marital stress were presented in session 6. Alteration of P's daily schedule to reduce stress during the times of the day when the flashes were most likely was worked on in session 7. Ps were given three trials of temperature biofeedback training . . . in session 8. [p. 138]**

Germaine and Freedman (1984) employed EEG biofeedback as a means of eliciting relaxation among a group of menopausal women. Biofeedback was not successful in producing a significant reduction in the frequency of reports of hot flashes.

For More Information

Germaine, L., & Freedman, R. (1984). Behavioral treatment of menopausal hot flashes: Evaluation by objective methods. *Journal of Consulting and Clinical Psychology, 52*, 1072-1079.

This article reports on the use of a procedure for assessing the menopausal hot flash. It also describes relaxation training with menopausal women. The article can be obtained from Leonard M. Germaine, Behavioral Medicine Laboratory, Lafayette Clinic, 951 E. Lafayette, Detroit, MI 48207.

Stevenson, D., & Delprato, D. (1983). Multiple component self-control program for menopausal hot flashes. *Journal of Behavior Therapy and Experimental Psychiatry, 14*, 137-140.

This article describes a multiple component and treatment program and its application to a sample of menopausal women. The program included relaxation training, thought stopping, and temperature biofeedback training. The article can be obtained from Dennis J. Delprato, Department of Psychology, Eastern Michigan University, Ypsilanti, MI 48197.

References

Germaine, L., & Freedman, R. (1984). Behavioral treatment of menopausal hot flashes: Evaluation by objective methods. *Journal of Consulting and Clinical Psychology, 52*, 1072-1079.

Stevenson, D., & Delprato, D. (1983). Multiple component self-control program for menopausal hot flashes. *Journal of Behavior Therapy and Experimental Psychiatry, 14*, 137-140.

27 Myopia

Assessment Strategies

Myopia is a disorder in which visual acuity of stimuli at far distances is impaired. Acuity may be measured by a number of tests. Collins, Epstein, and Hannay (1981) employed the Behavioral Acuity Test, the Bausch and Lomb Ortho-rater, and two eye charts. What follows is their description of these tests:

> **. . . the Behavioral Acuity Test . . . involves the presentation of letters and words of identical size to the training stimuli at four distances: 152.5 cm (5 ft.), 305 cm (10 ft.), 457.5 cm (15 ft.) and 610 cm (20 ft.). For the BAT-Letter assessment, 10 single letter stimuli (randomly selected from the 26 possible letters), were presented at each distance. Two three-letter and two six-letter words made up of letters identical to the training stimuli were presented at the same distances for the BAT-Word assessment.**
>
> **The Bausch and Lomb Ortho-rater was used to assess far distance binocular acuity. The Ortho-rater presents stimuli in a four-spatial-position forced-choice test, which provides reliable psychophysical measurements . . . and is a highly standardized visual screening device. . . . Acuity is assessed from 20/200 to 20/17 in 12 distinct steps.**
>
> **Two eye charts were also used. These were the Letter Chart for 20 ft. (Snellen Letter) and the Symbol Chart for 20 ft. (Snellen E). Each chart assesses acuity from 20/200 to 20/15 in eight distinct steps. [pp. 694-695]**

Treatment Strategies

Visual acuity may be improved in myopic patients through a behavioral training program employing a training procedure based on fading and verbal feedback (Epstein, Collins, Hannay, & Looney, 1978). The procedure is described as follows:

> **Subjects were instructed they would be shown letters of the alphabet at varying distances and asked to identify the letters shown. They were told that each stimulus would be presented for 5 sec, followed by a 5-sec rest. Glasses were removed right before the beginning of each training session. . . .**
>
> **The training stimuli were presented in random order, with the criterion for success at any distance being ten consecutive correct identifications. The stimuli were randomized by shuffling the stimulus cards every ten trials. . . . When the criterion was met, the distance from subject to stimulus was increased by 20 cm. [pp. 275-276]**

In applying this technique, social reinforcement by the therapist should follow each correct response.

Biofeedback has also been successfully used with myopic patients. Trachtman, Giambalvo, and Feldman (1981) employed a procedure in which an auditory tone was presented contingent on voluntary control of accommodation.

For More Information

Epstein, L., Collins, F., Hannay, H., & Looney, R. (1978). Fading and feedback in the modification of visual acuity. *Journal of Behavioral Medicine, 1*, 273-287.

This article describes two studies in which visual acuity was modified by gradually increasing the distance at which stimuli were discriminated and by providing verbal feedback on performance. Two measures of acuity are described. The article can be obtained from Leonard H. Epstein, Department of Psychiatry, Western Psychiatric Institute and Clinic, Pittsburgh, PA 15261.

References

Collins, F., Epstein, L., & Hannnay, H. (1981). A component analysis of an operant training program for improving visual acuity in myopic students. *Behavior Therapy, 12*, 692-701.

Epstein, L., Collins, F., Hannay, H., & Looney, R. (1978). Fading and feedback in the modification of visual acuity. *Journal of Behavioral Medicine, 1*, 273-287.

Trachtman, J., Giambalvo, V., & Feldman, J. (1981). Biofeedback of accommodation to reduce functional myopia. *Biofeedback and Self-Regulation, 6*, 547-562.

28 Neurodermatitis

Assessment Strategies

> **Neurodermatitis is a skin disorder characterized by circular, oval, or irregular patches of intensely pruritic, excessively furrowed and thickened shiny skin, except where covered by fine, gray scales. . . . These lesions are commonly seen in one or more of several classic locations, such as the elbows, knees, inner thighs, nape of neck, occipital area of the scalp, scrotum, vulva, the perianal region, eyelids, ears, and ankles. This disease begins with a small pruritic lesion or other minor irritation which incites a cycle of itching and scratching from which the chronic dermatosis develops. [Pinkerton, Hughes, & Weinrich, 1982, p. 249]**

A dermatological consultation should precede any behavioral assessment since neurodermatitis may be the result of physical causes, such as food allergies.

A behavioral assessment should include a daily frequency count of scratching for at least a one-week baseline. Some patients may require a wrist counter to aid in recording the behavior. Scratching can be objectively defined as "placing the hand on the affected area of the skin and scratching with the fingernails for at least 5 seconds" (Rosenbaum & Ayllon, 1981; p. 314). A separate frequency count of urges to scratch may be needed for some patients. Pictures of the affected areas can also be used as baseline measures. Additionally, anxiety should be assessed. A behavioral diary indicating the antecedants and consequences surrounding scratching episodes may be useful.

Treatment Strategies

Some patients may benefit from continued self-monitoring alone. This self-monitoring should include graphing the behavior on a daily basis. Extinction and reinforcement programs can easily be added to the self-monitoring. Instructions to ignore the scratching and not remark on it should be provided to significant persons in the patient's environment. Decreased frequency of scratching can be reinforced by the use of social or material reinforcers, or both, by significant others. Some patients may also be able to self-reinforce the decreased frequency. Reinforcement can also be applied by increasing behaviors incompatible with scratching (e.g., stroking the skin).

Rosenbaum and Ayllon (1981) have shown habit reversal to be very successful in treating the scratching behavior. They describe the procedure as follows:

> **The client verbally described and demonstrated scratching in the response description procedure. The first author then taught each client to detect bringing her hand toward the areas in which scratching occurred (e.g., ankle, arm, elbow) (*early warning*).**
>
> ***Situation awareness training* consisted of client descriptions of those situations in which scratching usually occurred or increased in frequency. Unpleasant aspects of scratching were described to increase the motivation to cease this behavior (*habit inconvenience review*).**

> **In the competing response practice procedure, each client was taught an isometric exercise characterized by: (a) being incompatible with scratching; (b) lasting at least one minute; (c) tensing the muscles used in scratching; (d) easy implementation with usual activities; and (e) preventing scratching from remaining a routine aspect of normal activities. The first author taught each client to place her hands in her lap or by the side of her body and clench her fists until a comfortable amount of tension was produced in the hands and forearms. This response was to be performed for 2 minutes following the urge to scratch, any antecedant to scratching or any occurrence of scratching. To relieve severe itching, each client was instructed to either stroke or pat the affected skin area. . . .**
>
> **In the *symbolic rehearsal* procedure, one situation in which scratching usually occurred was chosen. The client performed the competing response, as she recalled an actual instance of scratching in that situation. Following several repetitions of this procedure, the first author engaged the client in a general discussion. The client was instructed to perform the competing response whenever an urge to scratch, antecedent to scratching, or actual scratching occurred during this discussion. The first author pointed out any instances of scratching that the client failed to detect. The entire treatment session lasted about 60 minutes. [p. 315]**

If the assessment reveals that the scratching is precipitated by stressful situations, it may be necessary to utilize an anxiety reduction technique, such as relaxation training or systematic desensitization. Temperature biofeedback (Manuso, 1977) and frontal EMG biofeedback (Haynes, Wilson, Jaffe, & Britton, 1979) have also been used successfully to treat neurodermatitis.

For More Information

Rosenbaum, M. and Ayllon, T. (1981). The behavioral treatment of neurodermatitis through habit-reversal. *Behavioral Research and Therapy, 19*, 313-318.

This article describes the successful use of habit reversal treatment for dealing with scratching associated with neurodermatitis in four case studies. The article can be obtained from Michael S. Rosenbaum, Department of Pediatrics, University of South Alabama Medical Center, 2451 Fillingim Street, Mobile, AL 36617.

Watson, D., Tharp, R., & Crisberg, J. (1972). Case study in self-modification: Suppression of inflammatory scratching while awake and asleep. *Journal of Behavior Therapy and Experimental Psychiatry, 3*, 213-215.

This article describes the use of incompatible behaviors and self-reinforcement to reduce the scratching in a single case study. The article can be obtained from Roland, G. Tharp, Department of Psychology, University of Hawaii, Honolulu, HI 96822.

References

Haynes, S., Wilson, C., Jaffe, P., & Britton, B. (1979). Biofeedback treatment of atopic dermatitis: Controlled case studies of 8 cases. *Biofeedback and Self-Regulation, 4*, 195-209.

Manuso, J. (1977). The use of biofeedback assisted hand-warming training in the treatment of chronic eczematous dermatitis of the hands: A case study. *Journal of Behavior Therapy and Experimental Psychiatry, 8*, 445-446.

Pinkerton, S., Hughes, H., & Wenrich, W. (1982). *Behavior medicine clinical applications*. New York: John Wiley & Sons.

Rosenbaum, S., & Ayllon, T. (1981). Behavioral treatment of neurodermatitis through habit-reversal. *Behavior Research and Therapy, 19*, 313-318.

29 Pain — Acute

Assessment Strategies

Acute pain may be assessed on a number of dimensions. Pain ratings may be obtained from the patient. Postlewaite, Stirling, and Peck (1986) employed a five-point Likert rating scale to assess the average pain perceived over a 24-hour period. Patients used a similar scale to rate pain experienced during physical therapy.

More descriptive information on the patient's report of pain may be obtained by self-monitoring. Hamberger (1982) describes a procedure which includes spouse involvement:

> **The patient was initially instructed to self-monitor gastric pain attacks. The task involved providing a brief written description of situational variables, including physical setting, interpersonal interactions, and cognitions, in order to determine any possible relationship between psychosocial events and gastric attacks. The patient was also instructed to note the frequency and duration of the gastric attacks. The patient's wife was also instructed to monitor frequency and duration of discrete gastric attacks, independently of the patient, in a separate notebook. Frequency of gastric attacks was recorded by noting the date of onset of each attack. Duration was recorded by noting each complete day and night the patient remained in bed. Days-in-bed was defined as each 24-hr period of complete bedrest, except for brief periods out of bed for bathing and/or elimination. . . . During the first session, the nature and rationale of progressive relaxation as an active coping skill were presented. The patient was shown the specific procedure for tensing and relaxing each of 16 muscle groups, as recommended by Bernstein and Borkovec (1973). The patient was then taught to use feelings of tension as cues to begin relaxing (Goldfried & Trier, 1974). To facilitate training in active coping relaxation, the patient was taught to use his skill as an active coping response to specific imagined stressful situations. Examples of stressful scenes included unavoidable interpersonal conflicts, anger in response to frustration or failure in carrying out household maintenance tasks, and anxiety about returning for semiannual physical examinations. To augment the effects of the single "live" training session, the patient was provided with written didactic instructions in the use of active coping relaxation, as well as taped relaxation instructions. The patient was instructed to practice relaxation a minimum of once each day, and to apply the relaxation actively, as needed, in tense or stressful situations. [pp. 230-231]**

Fordyce, Brockway, Bergman, and Spengler (1986) used pain drawings to obtain information on the locus of pain.

Activity level may be used as an index of pain. Fordyce et al. (1986) describe a comprehensive assessment of activity level as follows:

> **The activity level was measured in two ways. First, 3 days of activity diary forms was completed by the S's at the time of follow-up. Those provided for recording the time spent sitting, standing/walking, and reclining by making four checks each hour to allocate the hour's time in quarter-hour units among those three body positions. Scoring consisted of the average number of checks recorded for each body position per day.The second activity level measure was the Activity Pattern Indicator (API) form. This is a checklist in which the person records the number**

of times the activity listed was engaged in in the week preceding completion of the form, in the case of probable higher-frequency activities (e.g., cooking, leaving the house for employment), or in the preceding month, for lower-probable frequency activities (e.g., banking). [p. 132]

Fordyce et al., (1986) also assessed "claimed impairment" in pain patients. This procedure is described as follows:

(1) Heaviest amount lifted (in pounds) in the preceding month.
(2) Longest interval sitting without having to stand in the preceding month.
(3) Longest interval standing without having to sit in the preceding month.
(4) Longest distance (in blocks) walked without having to stop to rest in the preceding month.
(5) Number of nights awakened by pain in the preceding week (used only at follow-up). [p. 131-132]

It is also possible to assess the patient's vocational status and health-care utilization. Fordyce et al. (1986) describe assessment of these areas as follows:

Vocational Status (V)

(1) Pain-derived income (Yes/No)
(2) Days not worked because of pain in the 30 days preceding follow-up.
(3) Days others helped with activities because of pain in the 30 days preceding follow-up.

Health-Care Utilization (HCU)

HCU Measures at Intake. These were as follows.
(1) Number of years in the preceding 20 in which professional help was sought for persisting pain.
(2) Number of different doctors or clinics visited during the preceding 10 years for pain.
(3) Number of surgeries for pain.
(4) Estimated amount spent by patient, insurance company, or health-care plan for pain medications in the past 6 months.
(5) Number of visits to doctor, house calls, and emergency-room visits for pain in the past 6 months.
(6) Were any such visits for back pain? (Yes/No)
(7) Number of hospitalizations for pain.

HCU Measures at Follow-Up. These were as follows.
(1) Since injury, the number of different treatments for back pain (e.g., traction, medications, massage).
(2) Since injury, the number of different doctors, clinics, or other professionals seen for back pain.
(3) Since injury, the number of visits to doctors, clinics, or other professionals for back pain.
(4) Estimated amount spent in preceding 30 days by patient, insurance company, or health-care plan for pain medications.
(5) Number of medications currently being taken for pain.
(6) Since injury, number of hospitalizations for pain.

[pp. 130-131]

Daily analgesic intake may also be assessed in the acute pain patient.

Finally, the clinician should assess levels of anxiety and depression as these may occur in the acute pain patient. Postlethwaite et al. (1986) employed the State-Trait Anxiety Inventory and the Depression Adjective Checklist as assessment instruments.

Treatment Strategies

Relaxation has been successfully employed as an active coping skill in acute pain. Hamberger (1982) taught an ostomy patient a modified version of Jacobson's progressive relaxation. The procedure is described as follows:

> **During the first session, the nature and rationale of progressive relaxation as an active coping skill were presented. The patient was shown the specific procedure for tensing and relaxing each of 16 muscle groups, as recommended by Bernstein and Borkovec (1973). The patient was then taught to use feelings of tension as cues to begin relaxing (Goldfried and Trier, 1974). To facilitate training in active coping relaxation, the patient was taught to use his skill as an active coping response to specific imagined stressful situations. Examples of stressful scenes included unavoidable interpersonal conflicts, anger in response to frustration or failure in carrying out household maintenance tasks, and anxiety about returning for semiannual physical examinations.**
>
> **To augment the effects of the single "live" training session, the patient was provided with written didactic instructions in the use of active coping relaxation, as well as taped relaxation instructions. The patient was instructed to practice relaxation a minimum of once each day, and to apply the relaxation actively, as needed, in tense or stressful situations.**
>
> **[p. 231]**

Fordyce et al., (1986) used a time-contingent behavioral program to successfully reduce acute back pain. Analgesics, if prescribed, were taken on a fixed-time interval schedule. Activity limits were specified by a physician and ended when a pre-set time interval elapsed. Exercises were performed with a pre-set number of repetitions and were increased at a physician's discretion.

Stress inoculation training has not been found to be effective with acute pain patients (Postlewaite, et al., 1986).

For More Information

Fordyce, W., Brockway, J., Bergman, J., & Spengler, D. (1986). Acute back pain: A control-group comparison of behavioral vs. traditional management methods. *Journal of Behavioral Medicine, 9*, 127-140.

This article describes a comprehensive assessment procedure and treatment program with a group of back pain patients. Assessment is conducted on a number of dimensions including locus of pain, activity level, and claimed impairment. This article can be obtained from Wilbert E. Fordyce, Rehabilitation Medicine, University of Washington, Seattle, WA 98195.

References

Fordyce, W., Brockway, J., Bergman, J., & Spengler, D. (1986). Acute back pain: A control-group comparison of behavioral vs.traditional management methods. *Journal of Behavioral Medicine, 9*, 127-140.

Hamberger, L., (1982). Reduction of generalized aversive responding in a post-treatment cancer patient: Relaxation as an active coping skill. *Journal of Behavior Therapy and Experimental Psychiatry, 13*, 229-233.

Postlethwaite, R., Stirling, G., & Peck, C. (1986). Stress inoculation for acute pain: A clinical trial. *Journal of Behavioral Medicine, 9*, 219-227.

See Also

Chapter 30. Pain - Chronic

30 Pain — Chronic

Assessment Strategies

Chronic pain has been defined as pain that persists for more than six months. Pain has also been considered chronic when appropriate medical intervention fails to provide relief, or when the intensity of pain is deemed disproportionate to the degree and type of disease or injury. Chronic pain is distinguished from acute pain as the latter is considered to be a symptom of disease or injury and is expected to be mitigated by appropriate medical treatment. Behavioral manifestations of chronic pain may include any of the following: verbal reports of pain, moaning, grimacing, limping, guarding the painful region, posturing, avoiding stimuli perceived as noxious, and displaying functional limitations (e.g., staying in bed for extended periods of time).

Assessment of chronic pain should include a general medical examination with orthopedic and neurological evaluations. The clinician should obtain a detailed patient history. The Cornell Medical Index (CMI) may be administered to the patient to assess bodily dysfunction and corresponding emotional status.

Information on topography of the region of pain and intensity and duration of pain from onset to present should be obtained. This information may be collected by interviewing thepatient. Reports from a family member are another source of information. Furthermore, the patient's display of pai behaviors may be observed by the clinican or by family members. Keefe and Brown (1982) describe an observation procedure implemented by hospital staff:

> **The observation procedure involved a nurse's observing the patient for five seconds every hour anad categorizing the patient's behavior in one of four categories: (a) pain behavior, (b) pain complaints—for example, talking about the pain; (c) in bed-for example, reclining in her room in bed or on the ward on a couch; or (d) "well behavior"—for example, involvement in recreational activities on the ward. [p. 29]**

Observations of pain behaviors may also be quantified by use of the UAB Pain Behavior Scale (Richards, Nepomuceno, Riles, & Suer, 1982) in which the observer rates frequency and severity of pain behaviors on a 3-point scale.

The clinician may also wish to use various paper and pencil measures in assessing the quality and intensity of the pain. The Haven-Yale Multidimensional Pain Inventory (MPI, Turk & Rudy, 1985) contains three parts. In the first part, patients rate the severity of their pain, how it interferes with their social and occupational functioning, how dissatisfied they are with their level of social and occupational functioning, the amount of support provided by significant others, the amount of control they feel they have over their life, and provide ratings of depression, irritability, and tension. The second part consists of patient ratings of how frequently, and by what methods (e.g., ignoring), other people respond to the patient's expression of pain. In the final part of the inventory the patient indicates any behaviors that are performed or not performed because of the pain.

The Pain Survey Schedule (Cautela, 1977) and the McGill Pain Questionnaire assess the patient's pain history. The Topographical Pain Representation (TPR) (Ransford, Cairns, & Mooney, 1976) is a useful measure of locus and description of pain. Pain intensity may be rated by the patient via a visual analog scale. In cases of low back pain, the Low Back Pain Questionnaire provides the clinician with pertinent information.

The clinician may use pain medication intake as an index of pain. Intake can be monitored by patient report or by observation. Activity level is another way to judge how pain is perceived by the patient. Activity level may be assessed by way of subjective report or by observation. The Daily Activity Schedule (DAS) is a form the patient uses to maintain a record of his activities hour by hour. Fordyce et al. (1973) employed a 10-point number scale, asking patients to rate degree of interference.

In lieu of activity level, the clinician may assess the amount of time per day that the patient is out of bed, the "up-time" (Cairns, Thomas, Mooney, & Pace, 1976). An up-time recorder may be used as a means of measuring this variable. The recorder is an apparatus attached to the patient's bed. It records and displays "up-time."

The patient's educational or vocational involvement may also be an important area to assess.

The MMPI may be administered to determine personality patterns of the chronic pain patient. It may also be useful in predicting whether intervention is likely to be sabotaged by the patient. Hudgens (1979) describes the mean MMPI profiles for a group of chronic pain patients as follows:

> **The "conversion V," or neurotic triad, with elevations on hypochondriasis, depression, and hysteria (scales 1,2,3) generally reflects the tendency to preoccupation with bodily functions and complaints. [p. 70]**

It is recommended that an evaluation of the patient's home, work, and other environments be conducted by a psychologist or social worker. The evaluation may be conducted by way of interview. Such an evaluation could provide the clinician with information regarding the factors that serve to maintain or promote pain behaviors. The clinician should assess the function of pain for the patient and the source(s) of reinforcement of pain behavior. Information may be obtained by interviewing the patient or family members, or both. The Psycho-Social Pain Inventory (PSPI) (Heaton et al., 1981) is a structured interview which was developed to assess these psychosocial aspects of pain.

Finally, both depression and anxiety may need to be assessed to treat many pain patients.

Treatment Strategies

Intervention programs based on principles of operant reinforcement have been used with success in treating chronic pain patients. A pain treatment program developed by Fordyce (1976) was applied to a population of hospitalized pain patients by Anderson, Cole, Gullickson, Hudgens, and Roberts (1977). The goals of the program were to decrease the frequency of pain behaviors and to increase the frequency of well behaviors. The program begins by administering all non-essential medication via a pain cocktail on a time-contingent basis. The pain cocktail is gradually reduced to zero ingredients of medicine. Concurrently, the patient's activity level is gradually increased. Family and staff are instructed in contingency management, described by Anderson et al. (1977) as follows:

> **The first 2 or 3 weeks are spent teaching the family members to identify pain behaviors and their responses to it, and learning to ignore all pain behaviors. As "well" behaviors appear in the patient's repertoire the family must learn to attend to these well behaviors. They do this by means of praise, encouragement and support and being attentive during periods of activity. . . . The staff ignores the patient's pain behaviors but appropriately rewards other kinds of interactions and activities of the patient. . . . The staff gives the patient reinforcement not only for activity, but also for the patient's progress in seeing him or herself as a responsible, adequate, functioning person once again. [p. 98]**

This type of intervention is used one to three times a week.

Keefe and Brown (1982) provided an outpatient contingency management intervention for a chronic pain patient who had successfully participated in an inpatient program.

> **An outpatient contingency management program was instituted prior to discharge. In this program, Mrs. B was asked to keep daily records of her own behavior, indicating the amount of time she spent standing, walking, sitting, or reclining. Goals in terms of activity were set for each week of outpatient treatment. Mrs. B was seen initially on a weekly, then a biweekly, and later a monthly basis. Arrangements were also made for Mrs. B to continue taking the pain cocktail mixture. [pp. 38-39]**

Redd (1982) successfully employed a time-out procedure contingent on crying. This included a differential social reinforcement schedule for behaviors incompatible with crying.

> **The sitter was instructed to interact with the patient normally; and at least once every 5 min, he was to go over to the patient's bed and ask him if he wanted anything. The sitter was also instructed that if the patient began to cry or moan, he was to check on the patient and correct any problems. However, if the patient continued to cry in the absence of any discernible problems, the sitter was to leave the room and remain outside as long as the patient was crying. . . . When the patient stopped crying the sitter was to wait 2 min before returning to the patient's room. [pp. 228-229]**

This procedure involved time out from social stimulation only. Patients did have access to other reinforcers (e.g., TV or books). All family and medical staff were instructed to use this time-out procedure any time they visited the patient.

Cairns, et al. (1976) report on an inpatient treatment program that employed a graphic display of activity level and up-time as a means of rewarding the patient for improvement.

> **Each bed on the unit is equipped with an "uptime" recorder. . . . Increases in walking distance and time on the exercycle are assigned daily by the physical**

> **therapist in the form of activity quotas. Quotas are posted each day on a quota board in the Physical Therapy Gym. Prior to beginning his daily program, the patient checks the quota board to learn the amount of walking and biking which he is to attempt that day. . . . Rounds are made . . . each day. . . . At this time, daily performance levels of walking distance and time on the exercycle are plotted and uptime is recorded. [p. 304]**

The information is displayed on a large graph near the patient's bed. Patients are given social reinforcement for improvement and are basically ignored if no improvement is noted.

Self-control techniques, including cognitive behavioral interventions and relaxation training, have also been successfully employed with chronic pain patients (e.g., Kerns, Turk, Holzman, & Rudy). Blinchik and Grzesiak (1979) treated pain patients with two cognitive strategies based on Meichenbaum's stress innoculation training.

> **The 1st step was to educate them regarding pain. To do this, they were provided with a conceptualization of pain using gate control concepts. . . . They were then trained to be aware of their thoughts, self-verbalizations, and self-instructions emitted prior to and/or during their experience of pain. They also were instructed to omit the word "pain" from their vocabularies and were trained in a "new cognitive representation of their pain experience" by using a set of self-descriptive statements when they felt pain: for example, "I feel aroused." . . . They were taught to employ a strategy that would involve them in a cognitive process that was related to, yet inconsistent with, the experience of pain . . . they were asked to role-play, they were encouraged to verbally reinforce themselves each time they used the procedure. Finally, it was stressed that what was learned in treatment was to be utilized between formal training sessions. [pp. 610-611]**

Relaxation training has been employed successfully with chronic pain patients in both inpatient and outpatient interventions.

Relaxation training is usually augmented by electromyographic (EMG) feedback. Keefe, Schapira, Williams, Brown, and Surwit (1981) report success in treating chronic low back pain patients with EMG-assisted relaxation training based on the program described by Wolpe and Lazarus (1966). Generalization of treatment gains was incorporated in the intervention.

> **In the initial training session, patients were instructed by a laboratory technician in an abbreviated form of progressive relaxation training. . . . Patients were also given an introduction to frontalis EMG biofeedback in the initial training session . . . technicians attached EMG electrodes and left the patient in a sound-attenuated laboratory chamber. . . . Tape recorded relaxation instructions were then played over the loudspeaker. After listening to the relaxation instructions, patients were immediately provided with EMG biofeedback. . . . Two steps were taken to facilitate transfer of relaxation skills from laboratory to other environments. First, patients were provided with a casette tape recording of relaxation instruction identical to that used in the laboratory and encouraged to practice with this tape a minimum of two times per day. Second, patients were given a packet of 1 cm. adhesive backed dots to be placed in their environment as cues for relaxation. Each time they saw a dot they were to scan major muscle groups for a full minute and relax these muscles as much as possible while still continuing with their routine activities. A frequency of 20-30 repetitions of this procedure per day was encouraged. [Keefe et al., 1981; p. 95]**

Grzesiak (1977) reports on the successful use of a relaxation meditation procedure described by French and Tupin (1974).

> **The simple relaxation technique is a relaxation-meditation procedure consisting of three successive components. First, the patient undergoes a sequence of muscle relaxation exercises to help him achieve respiratory and muscular relaxation.**
>
> **The patient is made comfortable, told to close his eyes, and led through a muscle relaxation sequence. He is told to concentrate on tensing and relaxing various muscle groups beginning with the hands and the upper extremities and then progressing through facial, neck, trunk, and lower extremity musculature. . . the second phase, the patient is instructed to let his mind drift gently and effortlessly to a memory or an image that is peaceful and relaxing. He is instructed to indicate, usually by lifting a finger, when his mind has captured such a memory or an image. . . . The third phase involves an effortless focusing of attention on the pleasant and relaxing memory or image. . . . The patient should remain relaxed for at least one minute before he is brought out of the altered, relaxed state. . . . Stress to the patient that he can learn and practice the relaxation procedure independent of the therapist.**
>
> **Also, the patient need not disclose the nature of his pleasant, relaxing memory. [Grzesiak, 1977; p. 270]**

Outpatient relaxation training interventions have also been reported to be successful in treating the chronic pain patient. Belar and Cohen (1979) describe a case study in which the patient was trained in EMG-assisted Jacobson progressive muscle relaxation with instructions to practice relaxation exercises at home at least twice daily for 20 minutes.

Relaxation training has also been employed in the treatment of phantom limb pain. Sherman et al. (1979) describe a case report of the use of EMG-assisted Jacobson relaxation training on eliminating phantom limb pain. EMG biofeedback has also been successfully used to reduce rheumatic back pain (Flor, Haas, Turk, & Koehler, 1983). Cognitive techniques have been successfully combined with biofeedback to treat pain in rheumatoid arthritic patients (Bradley, Young, Anderson, McDaniel, Turner, & Aguedelo, 1984).

> **Interventions that combine different treatment procedures are frequently used with chronic pain patients. A number of inpatient pain management programs have been developed. Morgan, Kremer, and Gaylor (1979) successfully combined contingency management, progressive muscular relaxation, and cognitive techniques.**
>
> **Seres and Newman (1976) describe a pain clinic which combines systematic reduction of analgesic medication, physical therapy, biofeedback, Jacobson's relaxation training, contingency management, and education classes that teach the patient about the mechanisms of chronic pain.**
>
> **Multidisciplinary treatment programs for outpatient rehabilitation have been successful in managing chronic pain. Khatami and Rush (1978) report on a program based on symptom control, stimulus control, and social system intervention.**
>
> **This first phase of therapy is designed to teach the patient how to modify the nature and severity of his pain. . . . Symptom control is designed to reverse this helpless and hopeless attitude by teaching the patient to master or control his pain. All patients received relaxation training with home practice or electromyographic biofeedback; one patient learned autohypnosis. . . . The specific techniques were adopted from the work of Beck,**

> **The patient identifies events which precipitate or exacerbate the pain and records the consequences of pain on personal, family and work satisfaction and activity. The patient records cognitions associated with increased pain and/or dysphoria. He/she learns to reappraise reality and correct these maladaptive, unrealistic cognitions, and the underlying misconceptions or beliefs during the sessions and all homework assignments. . . . Social system intervention consists of direct instructions to family members to modify the positive and negative reinforcers for pain behavior, or structured family therapy. . . . Non-pain behavior and autonomous functioning were also reinforced by therapist attention, while he attended less to pain-related behaviors. . . [pp. 163-165]**

Cautela (1977) reports on a treatment program based on covert conditioning and successfully employed with a chronic pain patient. Components of the intervention include thought stopping, relaxation, and covert reinforcement.

> **The client is told to yell, "Stop, relax" and then imagine a reinforcing scene every time he feels pain or the pain becomes more intense. He is told to continue this three part sequence until the pain subsides or is eliminated. Situations in which the pain occurs or is exacerbated are determined. Covert positive reinforcement is applied to these situations by having the client imagine he is in these situations and feels very comfortable and free from pain, and then he reinforces himself covertly. For example the client who reports he feels cramps when he wakes up in the morning is asked to imagine he wakes up feeling fine, comfortable and with no cramps, and then to imagine a pleasant scene. If at any time during the day or evening pain occurs or becomes more intense, the client is to imagine the situation again, but this time with no pain and with a reinforcing scene to follow. He is asked to do this five times for each pain event before retiring for the evening. As part of the therapeutic strategy, he is instructed not to complain about pain to anyone. Also, significant others are asked to ignore the client every time he complains of pain. If their cooperation is not obtained, the covert extinction procedure is employed . . . by which the client is asked to imagine that he is complaining of pain to someone but that that individual completely ignores him. If the pain is usually localized in a particular area of the body, he is especially trained to relax that part particularly intensely. [p. 49]**

Fordyce et al. (1973) included generalization training in their treatment package. They describe this training as follows:

> **Efforts to modify the natural environment of patients to encourage maintenance of treatment gains may be summarized under two general categories. The first category encompassed efforts to modify the spouse's response to pain and well behavior. The spouse was helped in interview training sessions to identify the patient's pain behavior, to identify his reactions to the patient's behavior, to identify well behaviors and his reactions to those, and to change his responses to those events in the desired and appropriate manner. . . . The second category included efforts to modify further the natural environment through facilitating the patient's re-entry into activities which had appeared to be reinforcing prior to onset of the pain problem. [p. 403]**

For More Information

Anderson, T., Cole, T., Gullickson, G., Hudgens, A., & Roberts, A. (1977) Behavior modification of chronic pain: A treatment program by a multidisciplinary team. *Clinical Orthopaedics and Related Research, 129*, 96-100.

This article describes an inpatient pain treatment program that includes family involvement. The patient's family and the hospital staff are instructed to attend to well behaviors while ignoring behaviors associated with the expression of pain. The article can be obtained from Thomas Anderson, M.D., Department of Physical Medicine and Rehabilitation, University of Minnesota.

Fordyce, W. (1976) Behavioral concepts in chronic pain and illness. In P. Davidson, (Ed.), *The behavioral management of anxiety, depression, and pain.* New York: Brunner/Mazel.

This chapter describes the development and maintenance of pain as an operant behavior. It also includes a behavioral analysis of chronic pain with a treatment and assessment protocol. The book can be obtained from Brunner/ Mazel, Inc., 64 University Place, New York, NY 10003.

Keefe, F., Gil, K., & Rose, S. (1986). Behavioral approaches in the multidisciplinary management of chronic pain: programs and issues. *Clinical Psychology Review, 6*, 87-113.

This article provides a review of multidisciplinary treatment programs based on behavior modification techniques and describes their application to chronic pain patients. It also describes the mechanisms of chronic pain. The article can be obtained from Frances J. Keefe, Department of Psychiatry, Duke University Medical Center, P.O. Box 3926, Durham, NC 27710.

Turk, D., & Rudy, T. (1987). Towards a comprehensive assessment of chronic pain patients. *Behavior Research and Therapy, 25*, 237-249.

This article discusses the behavioral assessment of pain, various self-report inventories and questionnaires, and comprehensive pain assessments that include medical, psychosocial, and behavioral modalities. The article can be obtained from Dennis Turk, Department of Psychiatry and Center for Pain Evaluation and Treatment, University of Pittsburgh School of Medicine, 230 Lothrop Street, Pittsburgh, PA 15213.

References

Anderson, T., Cole, T., Gullickson, G., Hudgens, A., & Roberts, A. (1977). Behavior modification of chronic pain: a treatment program by a multidisciplinary team. *Clinical Orthopedics and Related Research, 129*, 96-100.

Belar, C., & Cohen, J. (1979). The use of EMG feedback and progressive relaxation in the treatment of a woman with chronic back pain. *Biofeedback and Self-Regulation, 4*, 345-363.

Blinchik, E., & Grzesiak, R. (1979). Reinterpretive cognitive strategies in chronic pain management. *Archives of Physical Medical Rehabilitation, 60*, 609-612.

Bradley, L., Young, L., Anderson, K., McDaniel, L., Turner, R., & Aguedelo, C. (1984). Psychological approaches to the management of arthritis pain. *Social Science Medicine, 19*, 1353-1360.

Cairns, D., Thomas, L., Mooney, V., & Pace, J. (1976). A comprehensive treatment approach to chronic low back pain. *Pain, 2*, 201-300.

Cautela, J. (1977). The use of covert conditioning in modifying pain behavior. *Journal of Behavior Therapy and Experimental Psychiatry, 8*, 45-52.

Flor, H., Hagg, G., Turk, D., & Koehler, H. (1983). Efficacy of EMG biofeedback pseudotherapy and conventional medical treatment for chronic rheumatic back pain. *Pain, 17*, 21-31.

Fordyce, W. (1976). Behavioral concepts in chronic pain and illness. In P. Davidson, (Ed.), *The behavioral management of anxiety, depression, and pain*. New York: Brunner/Mazel.

Fordyce, W., Fowler, R., Lehmann, J., DeLateur, B., Sand, P., & Trieschmann, R. (1973). Operant conditioning in the treatment of chronic pain. *Archives of Physical Medical Rehabilitation, 54*, 399-408.

French, A., & Tupin, J. (1974). Therapeutic application of a simple relaxation method. *American Journal of Psychotherapy, 28*, 282-287.

Grzesiak, R. (1977). Relaxation techniques in treatment of chronic pain. *Archives of Physical Medical Rehabilitation, 58*, 270-272.

Heaton, R., Getto, C., Lehman, R., Fordyce, W., Brauer, E., & Froban, S. (1981). Standardized evaluation of psychosocial factors in chronic pain. *Pain, 12*, 165-174.

Hudgens, A. (1979). Family-oriented treatment of chronic pain. *Journal of Marital and Family Therapy, 5*(4), 67-78.

Keefe, F., & Brown, C. (1982). Behavioral treatment of chronic pain syndromes. In P. Boudewyns & F. Keefe (Eds.), *Behavioral medicine in general medicine practice* (pp. 19-41) Reading, MA: Addison-Wesley.

Keefe, F., Schapira, B., Williams, R., Brown, C., & Surwit, R. (1981). EMG-assisted relaxation training in the management of chronic low back pain. *American Journal of Clinical Biofeedback, 4*, 93-103.

Kerns, R., Turk, D., Holzman, A., & Rudy, T. (1986). Comparison of cognitive-behavioral and behavioral approaches to the outpatient treatment of chronic pain. *Clinical Journal of Pain, 1*, 199-203.

Kerns, R., Turk, D., & Rudy, T. (1985). The West Haven-Yale Multidimensional Pain Inventory (WHYMPI). *Pain, 23*, 345-356.

Khatami, M., & Rush, A. (1978). A pilot study of the treatment of outpatients with chronic pain: Symptom control, stimulus control and social system intervention. *Pain, 5*, 163-172.

Morgan, C., Kremer, E., & Gaylor, M. (1979). The behavioral medicine unit: A new facility. *Comprehensive Psychiatry, 20*, 79-89.

Ransford, A., Cairns, D., & Mooney, V. (1976). The pain drawing as an aid in the psychologic evaluation of patients with low-back pain. *Spine, 1*, 127-134.

Redd, W. (1982). Treatment of excessive crying in a terminal cancer patient: A time-series analysis. *Journal of Behavioral Medicine, 5*, 225-235.

Richards, Nepomuceno, C., Riles, M., & Suer, Z., (1982). Assessing pain behavior: The UAB Pain Behavior Scale. *Pain, 14*, 393-398.

Seres, J., & Newman, R. (1976). Results of treatment of chronic low-back pain at the Portland Pain Center. *Journal of Neurosurgery, 45*, 32-36,

Sherman, R., Gall, N., & Gormly, J. (1979). Treatment of phantom limb pain with muscular relaxation training to disrupt the pain-anxiety-tension cycle. *Pain, 6*, 47-35.

Wolpe, J., & Lazarus, A. (1966). *Behavior therapy techniques.* New York, NY: Pergamon Press.

See Also

Chapter 29. Pain - Acute

31 Raynaud's Disease

Assessment Strategies

Raynaud's disease is a "functional disorder of the cardiovascular system in which the patient experiences painful episodes of vasoconstriction in the hands, and possibly the feet, which leave the extremities cold to the touch" (Blanchard & Haynes, 1975, p. 230). During a vasospasm attack, the digits of the hands or feet, or both, change colors, going from a blanching whiteness to a blue color, as oxygen reaching the fingers is reduced, and finally to a red color as oxygenated blood spreads within the digits. These coloration changes are due to vasospasms and may last for minutes or for hours. A rheumatological consultation should precede a behavioral assessment. Vasospasms may be due to scleroderma, connective tissue disease, lupus erythematosus, or other vascular diseases.

Behavioral assessment should include a daily record of vasospastic attacks. Keefe (1982) has developed an excellent behavioral log (see Table 31-1) to record both frequency and severity of attacks.

Keefe (1982) suggests that this baseline should continue for four weeks to increase the patient's awareness of any pattern of vasospastic attacks.

A cold stress test can be an excellent behavioral measure of a patient's ability to control digital skin temperature. However, this test requires a specially designed chamber capable of manipulating temperature.[1] Administration of the Psychological Screening Inventory (Nanyon, 1973) can help predict which Raynaud's disease patients will respond well to autogenic training.

Anxiety should also be assessed. Expanding the behavioral diary of vasospastic attacks to include the antecedents of anxiety and SUDS ratings of anxiety may be useful for many patients.

Treatment Strategies

For idiopathic Raynaud's disease a home program of autogenic training or progressive muscle relaxation may be the easiest intervention to initiate. Patients who score low on the alienation scale of the psychological screening inventory do well with autogenic training. Surwit and Fenton (1980) have used the following autogenic training instructions for heaviness:

> **I feel quiet. I am beginning to feel quite relaxed. My right foot feels heavy and relaxed. My left foot feels heavy and relaxed. My ankles, knees, and hips feel heavy, relaxed and comfortable. My abdomen and chest feel heavy and relaxed. My neck, jaw, and forehead feel completely relaxed. They feel comfortable and smooth. My right arm feels heavy and relaxed. My left arm feels heavy and relaxed. My right hand feels heavy and relaxed. My left hand feels heavy and relaxed. Both of my hands feel heavy and relaxed. Repeat to yourself, "My hands feel heavy and relaxed." [p. 130]**

---

[1] Available from The Psychological Corporation, 757 Third Ave., New York, NY 10017.

Table 31-1 Sample log used to record vasospastic attacks

Week of: ____________

	No. of attacks	Severity	Area	Side	Temperature	Home practice		
Monday						AM	Beg.	End
						PM	Beg.	End
Tuesday						AM	Beg.	End
						PM	Beg.	End
Wednesday						AM	Beg.	End
						PM	Beg.	End
Thursday						AM	Beg.	End
						PM	Beg.	End
Friday						AM	Beg.	End
						PM	Beg.	End
Saturday						AM	Beg.	End
						PM	Beg.	End
Sunday						AM	Beg.	End
						PM	Beg.	End

Severity
0 = No problem at all
1 = Mild disturbance—that is, cold hands, cold feet
2 = Uncomfortable; one or more blanched digits
3 = Moderate attack; painful, numb
4 = Very painful; one or more blanched digits
5 = Extremely painful; similar to the most severe attack you have ever had

Area: Area of attack
H = Hand
FT = Foot
F = Face

Side: Side of body
L = Left
R = Right
B = Both

Temperature: Outside temperature

Below 0°	50°s
0°	60°s
10°s	70°s
20°s	80°s
30°s	90°s
40°s	100°s

Keefe, 1982; p.156

Patients then hear a tone every 15 seconds and repeat the phrase "My hands feel heavy and relaxed" after each tone.

Surwit and Fenton (1980) gave patients a different set of instructions, emphasizing warmth, the second week:

> **I feel quiet. My whole body is relaxed and comfortable. My right arm is heavy and warm. My left arm is heavy and warm. My right hand is becoming warmer. My left hand is becoming warmer. Warmth is flowing into my hands. They are warm. I can feel the warmth flowing down into my right hand. It is warm and relaxed. I can feel the warmth flowing down into my left hand. It is warm and relaxed. My hands are warm and heavy. Repeat to yourself, "My hands are warm and heavy." Approximately every 15 seconds you will hear a tone. When you hear the tone, repeat to yourself, "My hands are warm and heavy, my hands are warm and heavy." [p. 130]**

Patients are instructed to practice two times per day at home, using the cassette tape of the instructions. After the patients have mastered the autogenic training via tapes, they can be instructed to practice warming their hands without the tapes for 30 to 60 seconds, 20 to 30 practice times per day. It may be helpful to cue the practice by associating various activities with hand-warming (e.g., going into a certain room or eating meals).

Some patients have difficulty generalizing the behavior to a wide variety of situations. Keefe (1982) suggests that the patient set up a stimulus hierarchy. The "hierarchy can range from the least difficult practice situation (for example, in a warm room) all the way up to the most difficult training situation (such as grabbing a cold door knob). The patients can then begin practicing in the least difficult situation and gradually work their way up to more difficult training situations" (p. 162). Improvement should be seen very rapidly (in 7 to 10 days) with the use of these techniques.

Progressive muscle relaxation training has also been found to be effective for treatment of Raynaud's disease (Jacobson, Manschreck, & Silverberg, 1979).

Autogenic training and relaxation training generally are as effective as biofeedback approaches (Jacobson et al., 1979; Surwit, Pilon, & Fenton, 1978).

An inexpensive biofeedback instrument can be added to the autogenic training or relaxation training programs. A small liquid crystal thermometer with adhesive backing can be attached to the patient's middle finger to serve as a simple temperature biofeedback device. The thermometer is called a physiologic trend indicator.[2]

If the assessment reveals that anxiety is an antecedent to vasospastic attacks, it may be necessary to apply anxiety reduction techniques, such as systematic desensitization.

Fingertip skin temperature biofeedback has been found to be successful in treating Raynaud's disease (Blanchard & Hayes, 1975; Surwit, 1973; May & Weber, 1976). The addition of biofeedback training under cold stress tends to maintain gains over time (Freedman, Ianni, & Wenig, 1983). Feedback may also be helpful for treating Raynaud's phenomena secondary to other disorders. May and Weber (1976) and Freedman, Ianni, Hale, and Lynn (1979) used skin temperature biofeedback to treat Raynaud's phenomena secondary to scleroderma.

---

[2] The thermometer can be obtained from the Medical Device Corporation, Indianapolis, IN.

However, the effects may not persist on long term followup (Freedman, Ianni, & Wenig, 1984). Keefe, Surwit, and Pilon (1978) used biofeedback to treat a patient suffering from Raynaud's phenomena secondary to mixed connective tissue disease.

The addition of a cognitive stress management approach to autogenic training, or biofeedback, does not enhance the treatment effects (Freedman, Ianni, & Wenig, 1983).

A classical conditioning treatment, using a cold chamber, has been found to be effective (Jobe, Sampson, Roberts, & Kelly, 1986).

For More Information

Keefe, F. (1982). Behavioral treatment of Raynaud's disease. In P. Boudewyns & F. Keefe (Eds.), *Behavioral medicine in general medical practice* (pp. 145-165). Menlo Park, CA: Addison-Wesley.

This chapter describes the physiology and pathophysiology of Raynaud's disease. Medical and surgical treatment as well as behavioral approaches to treatment are reviewed. There is an excellent description of a behavioral assessment and treatment program for Raynaud's disease, incorporating both autogenic training and biofeedback procedures. The book can be obtained from Addison-Wesley Publishing Co., 1 Jacob Way, Reading, MA 01867.

Surwit, R. (1981). Behavioral approaches to Raynaud's disease. *Psychotherapy Psychosomatics, 36*, 224-245.

This excellent review article covers the description and diagnosis of the disorder, medical treatment, biofeedback and behavioral treatment approaches. The article can be obtained from Richard Surwit, Department of Psychiatry, Duke University Medical Center, Box 3842, Durham, NC 27710.

Surwit, R., Pilon, R., & Eaton, C. (1978). Behavioral treatment of Raynaud's disease. *Journal of Behavioral Medicine, 1*, 323-334.

This article describes the successful use of autogenic training and a combination of autogenic training and skin temperature biofeedback in treating 30 Raynaud's disease patients. There is a good description of the cold stress test and programming for generalization of treatment effects. The article can be obtained from Richard Surwit, Department of Psychiatry, Duke University Medical Center, Box 3842, Durham, NC 27710.

References

Blanchard, E., & Haynes, M. (1975). Biofeedback treatment of a case of Raynaud's disease. *Journal of Behavior Therapy and Experimental Psychiatry, 6*, 230-234.

Freedman, R., Ianni, P., Hale, P., & Lynn, S. (1979). Treatment of Raynaud's phenomena with biofeedback and cold desensitization. *Psychophysiology, 16*, 182.

Freedman, R., Ianni, P., & Wenig, P. (1983). Behavioral treatment of Raynaud's disease. *Journal of Consulting and Clinical Psychology, 51*, 539-549.

Freedman, R. Ianni, P., & Wenig, P. (1984). Behavioral treatment of Raynaud's phenomenon in scleroderma. *Journal of Behavioral Medicine, 7,* 343-353.

Jacobson, A., Manschreck, T., & Silverberg, E. (1979). Behavioral treatment for Raynaud's disease: A comparative study with long-term followup. *American Journal of Psychiatry, 136*, 844-846.

Jobe, J., Sampson, J., Roberts, D., & Kelly, J. (1986). Comparison of behavioral treatments for Reynaud's disease. *Journal of Behavioral Medicine, 9*, 89-96.

Keefe, F. (1982). Behavioral treatment of Raynaud's disease. In P. Boudewyns & F. Keefe (Eds.), *Behavioral medicine in general medical practice* (pp. 145-165). Menlo Park, CA: Addison-Wesley.

Keefe, F., Surwit, R., & Pilon, R. (1978, November). Collagen-vascular disease: Can behavior therapy help? Paper presented at the meeting of the Association of the Advancement of Behavior Therapy, Chicago, IL.

Lanyon, R. (1973). *Psychological Screening Inventory: Manual.* Goshen, NY: Research Psychologists.

Nay, D., & Weber, C. (1976). Temperature feedback training for symptom reduction in primary and secondary Raynaud's disease. *Biofeedback and Self-Regulation, 1*, 317.

Surwit, R. (1973). Biofeedback: A possible treatment for Raynaud's disease. *Seminars in Psychiatry, 5*, 483-490.

Surwit, R., & Fenton, C. (1980). Feedback and instructions in the control of digital skin temperature. *Psychophysiology, 17*, 129-132.

Surwit, R., Pilon, R., & Fenton, C. (1978). Behavioral treatment of Raynaud's disease. *Journal of Behavior Medicine, 1*, 323-335.

32 Seizure Disorder

Assessment Strategies

Seizure disorders are central nervous system disorders characterized by abnormal EEG activity and resultant interruptions in sensory, motor, or cognitive functions. The origin of seizure disorders may be organic or psychogenic.

The International Classification of Epileptic Seizures (Gastaut, 1970) provides a system of categorizing the disorders on the basis of behavioral manifestations and EEG activity.

Assessment of seizure disorders should include a detailed history of seizures. Age at onset, frequency and duration, and description of behavioral manifestations of seizures may be obtained through an interview with the patient or family. The clinician should assess whether the occurrence of seizures is associated with, or triggered by, specific environmental stimuli. A family history should also be obtained.

In addition to a general physical evaluation, a neurological examination, including an EEG, is necessary. Neuropsychological testing may be conducted to determine presence and severity of impairment.

It may also be important to evaluate the patient's depression, since many seizure patients experience significant depression (Davis, Armstrong, Donovan, & Temkin, 1984).

Treatment Strategies

Procedures based on respondent conditioning (e.g., extinction or habituation) have been successfully used in the treatment of seizure disorders. In some cases of epilepsy, seizures are induced by exposure to specific stimuli. For example, patterns of sound or melodies may precipitate a seizure in cases of musicogenic epilepsy. Certain light frequencies will induce seizures in stroboscopic epilepsy. In cases of reading epilepsy, the seizure occurs in response to the activity of reading.

Extinction procedures have been used to render the noxious stimulus innocuous. Forster, Booker, and Gascon (1967) describe the procedure as applied to musicogenic epileptics:

> **These newer techniques consisted of the continuous playing of the noxious number despite the appearance of spiking dysrhythmia in the EEG. With repeated presentations the electroencephalographic abnormality diminished and finally disappeared and the musical number became innocuous. . . . Reinforcement tapes were prepared for each patient. These tapes consisted of the music which had been noxious, either producing a seizure or EEG dysrhythmia in our laboratory, and to which the patient had been repeatedly exposed until this number became innocuous. These reinforcement tapes are audited twice daily by the patients. [p. 236]**

Conditioning therapy has been used successfully in cases of reading epilepsy. Forster, Paulsen, and Baughman (1969) employed two methods of conditioning with a patient. They describe these procedures as follows:

> **The first method chosen for conditioning was the use of vigilance techniques for maintaining the patient's concentration during the reading of the Gettysburg Address. He was, therefore, instructed to tap his thigh each time he saw the articles "the" and "a." . . . The choice . . . shifted to an alphabet letter . . . was told to pat his thigh each time a letter "a" occurred. This was done with"a" and later with "e." . . . This was then changed to tapping with the fingers rather than his hand, then simply pressing his fingers together when he saw the particular letters. Reading without the attention to the alphabet promptly evoked a discharge again. He was returned to the alphabet for more trials and afterward he was able, on consecutive trials, to read the Gettysburg Address without particular attention to vowels and without a dysrhythmia. . . . A second method of conditioning was also developed for the patient. He was given a new passage . . . and told to read it quietly several times without moving his lips, then merely moving his lips inaudibly, and finally aloud, and this was done without evocation of seizures or dysrhythmias. [pp. 719-720]**

Procedures based on principles of operant conditioning have been used with success in the treatment of seizure disorders. Cautela and Flannery (1973) delivered reinforcement contingent on seizure-free periods and withheld reinforcement when seizures occurred. They describe the procedure as follows:

> **Each day the teacher-therapist told Mr. C. that if he did not have a seizure that day, she would spend some time talking to him. And during the day, social praise and candy were given to him. Conversely, if the client had a seizure, another staff member assisted the patient only enough to prevent injury. No staff talking was permitted during or just after the seizure. The authors knew of only one set of antecedent stimuli to correlate with seizures, the mention of doctors or hospitals. The teachers were instructed to avoid the use of those words or a discussion of related issues in class. Also, the teachers were told to continually assess the client's behavior for more antecedent stimuli and for possible reinforcers. [pp. 34-35]**

Iwata and Lorentzson (1976) developed a program that included increased daily activities, differential reinforcement of other behavior, and time-out contingent on seizures.

Relaxation may also be employed as an intervention for seizure disorders. Wells, Turner, Bellack, and Hersen (1978) describe an application of cue-controlled relaxation to the management of seizures:

> **One session of therapist administered and two sessions of self-administered relaxation training occurred daily. Once a state of deep relaxation was obtained, the therapist and patient (in concert) vocalized the cue word "relax" 25 times during exhalation. Finally, the patient was instructed to vividly imagine five situations involving pre-seizure auras and subsequent seizure activity that had taken place on the unit. Following the patient's signal (raised finger) that she was clearly imagining her premonitory symptoms (i.e., the aura) the therapist said "relax"until a deep state of relaxation was once again achieved. The patient was asked to subvocalize this cue word along with the therapist. . . . Also, the patient was instructed to employ the cue word during pre-seizure auras on the unit. [p. 51]**

EEG biofeedback has occasionally been used successfully in the treatment of seizure disorders (e.g., Steman & Friar, 1973). Typically, patients are instructed to relax and to think whatever thoughts are necessary to achieve a mental state conducive to inhibition of seizures. Biofeedback may be combined with verbal or monetary rewards to enhance motivation.

Procedures may be combined in order to maximize the effectiveness of treatment. Daniels (1975) developed a program that included operant techniques and covert conditioning in the treatment of seizures.

> **. . . it became clear the environmental contingencies were maintaining the behavior. Covert extinction was again applied. . . . In addition, all staff and clients were instructed to ignore her seizure episodes. Behavior modification training with staff members and co-workers required that following each seizure they make no conversation and not assist her in changing soiled clothing caused by incontinence and falling. A point system was also introduced that allowed her to earn points for such low probability behaviors as not having a seizure, taking prescribed medications on time, weight loss, social and recreational excursions with friends, using publictransportation, dating, and cooking meals at home for her family. Accumulated points were exchangeable for opportunities to work as a hairdresser. [p. 66]**

For More Information

Forster, F., Hansotia, P., Cleeland, C., & Ludwig, A. (1969). A case of voice-induced epilepsy treated by conditioning. *Neurology, 19*, 325-331.

This article describes the treatment of voice-induced epilepsy with conditioning therapy. The article can be obtained from: Francis M. Forster, M.D., Department of Neurology, University Hospitals, University of Wisconsin Medical Center, 1300 University Avenue, Madison, WI 53706.

Lowman, R., & Richardson, L. (1987). Pseudoepileptic seizures of psychogenetic origin: A review of the literature. *Clinical Psychology Review, 7*, 363-389.

This article thoroughly reviews the nature and history of the disorder, epidemiological findings, diagnosis, assessment procedures, etiology, and the behavioral interventions of relaxation and environmental manipulations. The article can be obtained from Rodney Lowman, Division of Occupational Medicine, Duke University Medical Center, Box 2914, Durham, NC 27710.

Mostofsky, D., & Balaschak, B. (1977). Psychobiological control of seizures. *Psychological Bulletin, 84*, 723-750.

This article provides a review of behavioral treatment procedures used in the management of seizure disorders. Procedures include reward and punishment programs, self-control, and psychophysiological techniques. The article can be obtained from David I. Mostofsky, Department of Psychology, Boston University, Boston, MA 02215.

References

Cautela, J., & Flannery, R. (1973). Seizures: Controlling the uncontrollable. *Journal of Rehabilitation, 39*, 34-39.

Daniels, L. (1975). Treatment of grand mal epilepsy by covert and operant conditioning techniques: A case study. *Psychosomatics, 16*, 65-67.

Davis, G., Armstrong, H., Donovan, D., & Temkin, N. (1984). Cognitive-behavioral treatment of depressed affect among epileptics: Preliminary findings. *Journal of Clinical Psychololgy, 40*, 930-935.

Efron, R. (1956). The effect of olfactory stimuli in arresting uncinate fits. *Brain, 79*, 267-281.

Forster, F., Booker, H., & Gascon, G. (1967). Conditioning in musicogenic epilepsy. *Transactions of the American Neurological Association, 92*, 236-237.

Forster, F., Hansotia, P., Cleeland, C., & Ludwig, A. (1969).A case of voice-induced epilepsy treated by conditioning. *Neurology, 19*, 319-325.

Forster, F., Paulsen, U., & Baughman, F. (1969). Clinical therapeutic conditioning in reading epilepsy. *Neurology, 19*, 717-723.

Gastaut, H. (1970). Clinical and electroencephalographic classification of epileptic seizures. *Epilepsia, 11*, 102-113.

Iwata, B., & Lorentzson, A. (1976). Operant control of seizure-like behavior in an institutionalized retarded adult. *Behavior Therapy, 7*, 247-251.

Mostofsky, D., & Bataschak, B. (1977). Psychobiological control of seizures. *Psychological Bulletin, 84*, 723-750.

Sterman, M., & Friar, L. (1972). Supression of seizures in an epileptic following sensorimotor EEG feedback training. *Electroencephalography and Clinical Neurophysiology, 33*, 89-95.

Wells, K., Turner, S., Bellack, A., & Hersen, M. (1978). Effects of cue-controlled relaxation on psychomotor seizures: An experimental analysis. *Behavior Research and Therapy, 16*, 51-53.

33 Spasmodic Torticollis

Assessment Strategies

Spasmodic torticollis is a movement disorder characterized by the involuntary movement of the head. Usually the head is rotated to one side. Because there can be both organic and psychological causes for this disorder, it is important that any psychological treatment be preceded by a medical and neurological evaluation. One guideline in determining the etiology is the mode of onset of the disorder. If there is a sudden onset, the disorder is more likely to be psychological, and if there is a gradual onset, an organic basis should be suspected.

Behavioral assessment can involve ratings by both the patient and the therapist on a number of variables. These include: 1) amount of head movement, 2) regularity of movement, 3) degree of head tilt, 4) presence of spasms, 5) how noticeable the spasms are, and 6) the level of social disruption the spasms would likely produce. Each of these variables can be rated on a seven-point Likert Scale with "1" being none and "7" extreme.

Additionally, an assessment of the patient's general level of anxiety (e.g., State-Trait Anxiety Inventory), or a SUDS rating, can be helpful.

Treatment Strategies

There are three different behavioral techniques that have been successful in the treatment of spasmodic torticollis. For patients who demonstrate a high level of anxiety, the approach of systematic desensitization may be useful. The following three hierarchies are suggested by Meares (1972): 1) A temporal hierarchy. The patient is asked to imagine various head positions at times in the future and to signal whether or not a particular situation provoked anxiety. The distance into the future is then steadily decreased; 2) A hierarchy of imagined head position. The patient is asked to imagine his head in various degrees of deviation in the present; 3) A hierarchy of desensitization in practice. The head is moved less than the angle of deviation which arouses anxiety in fantasy. Initially the therapist, and later the patient himself, moves the head.

The second technique consists of an operant conditioning program using a metronome. Erickson and Huber (1975) describe the procedure as follows:

> **The procedure basically consisted of having the patient make small head movements in synchronization with the beat of a metronome. This was accomplished by having the patient, while sitting in a chair in the middle of his room, fixate a reference point on the wall. This reference point was centered in his visual field with his neck in the tonic position. Starting from this fixation point, which served as the referent visual stimulus, the patient made a slight head turn to the right so as to center his gaze upon a target visual stimulus. The target stimulus was placed approximately one foot to the right of the reference visual stimulus, along the wall. The visual stimuli were placed vertically on the wall at eye level, and consisted of six inch strips of tape. Therefore, with each beat of the metronome the patient turned his head from the referent visual stimulus to the target visual stimulus, and**

> **back again, thus completing a head turn to the right. Since the patient was seated approximately five feet from the wall, each of these head turns subtended a small angle (about five degrees) of rotation. The target visual stimulus was moved horizontally one foot farther to the right from the fixed reference visual stimulus every two days. Thus, the target stimulus was gradually moved along the walls of the patient's room, at increasing distances from the fixed reference stimulus until a head turn of 180 degrees was accomplished. The patient's head turning proceeded at the rate of 40 beats/minute as determined by the metronome setting. He also was instructed to turn off the metronome and cease head turning for a period of five minutes, whenever he encountered great pain or spasms during the training sessions. The patient practiced this procedure for two ten minute training periods per day. [pp. 405-406]**

Negative feedback has been used somewhat successfully by utilizing a bright light as a signal to the patient whenever torticollis occurs. The addition of instructions to the patient does not increase the effectiveness of the negative feedback.

Massed practice has been used with mixed results. The massed practice generally consists of having the patient voluntarily imitate the head movement rapidly and continuously for a set amount of time. If massed practice is attempted, a large number of trials per session (as many as 400) should be used. It is also important that the patient be able to return his head to a "normal" position during massed practice trials.

Both electrical aversion therapy (Brierly, 1967) and EMG biofeedback (Jones, Massong, & Buckley, 1983) have also been demonstrated to be effective for some patients with this disorder. Cleeland (1973) combined EMG biofeedback with contingent shock to reduce the spasm frequency in eight of ten patients. Additionally, Harrison, Garrett, Henderson, and Adams (1985) successfully used a device that provided auditory or visual feedback contingent on forward or lateral head tilt.

For More Information

Bernhardt, A., Hersen, M., & Barlow, D. (1972). Measurement and modification of spasmodic torticollis: An experimental analysis. *Behavior Therapy, 3*, 294-297.

This article describes the technique of negative feedback in a case study. A more sophisticated assessment device that requires a videotape monitor is also described. The article can be obtained from Michael Hersen, Department of Psychiatry, WPIC, 3811 O'Hara Street, Pittsburgh, PA 15261.

Meares, R. (1973). Behavior therapy in spasmodic torticollis. *Archives of General Psychiatry, 28*, 104-107.

This article reviews the previously attempted treatments for spasmodic torticollis and describes the successful treatment of one patient by using systematic desensitization. The article can be obtained from Russell Meares, M.D., Department of Psychiatry, University of Melbourne, Heidelberg, Victoria, 3084, Australia.

References

Brierly, H. (1967). The treatment of hysterical spasmodic torticollis by behavior therapy. *Behavior Research and Therapy, 5*, 139-142.

Cleeland, C. (1973). Behavioral techniques in the modification of spasmodic torticollis. *Neurology, 23*, 1241-1247.

Ericksen, R., & Huber, H. (1975). Elimination of hysterical torticollis through the use of a metronome in an operant conditioning paradigm. *Behavior Therapy, 6*, 405-406.

Harrison, D., Garrett, J., Henderson, D., & Adams, H. (1985). Visual and auditory feedback for head tilt and torsion in a spasmodic torticollis patient. *Behavior Research and Therapy, 23*, 87-88.

Jones, G., Massong, S., & Buckley, M. (1983). Treatment of spasmodic torticollis through spasm control and muscle reeducation: A case study. *Behavior Therapy, 13*, 178-184.

Meares, R. (1973). Behavior therapy in spasmodic torticollis. *Archives of General Psychiatry, 28*, 104-107.

34 Tardive Dyskinesias

Assessment Strategies

Many patients who have taken neuroleptic medication develop involuntary movements of the facial area (e.g., smacking movements of the lips), limbs, or trunk. These stereotype movements are called tardive dyskinesias. Any behavioral assessment of this disorder should be preceded by a thorough neurological evaluation. After objectively defining each movement, an initial behavioral assessment can involve a time-sampled frequency count of each of the movements. Additionally, a global rating scale, such as the Abnormal Involuntary Movement Scale[1] (AIMS), is available for the therapist and significant other to rate the severity of the movements. The examination procedure used for determining the ratings is shown in Table 34-1.

Table 34-1

EXAMINATION PROCEDURE FOR AIMS

Either before or after completing the Examination Procedure observe the patient unobtrusively, at rest (e.g., in waiting room).

The chair to be used in this examination should be a hard, firm one without arms.

1. Ask patient whether there is anything in his/her mouth (i.e., gum, candy, etc.) and if there is, to remove it.

2. Ask patient about the *current* condition of his/her teeth. Ask patient if he/she wears dentures. Do teeth or dentures bother patient *now*?

3. Ask patient whether he/she notices any movements in mouth, face, hands, or feet. If yes, ask to describe and to what extent they *currently* bother patient or interfere with his/her activities.

4. Have patient sit in chair with hands on knees, legs slightly apart, and feet flat on floor. (Look at entire body for movements while in this position.)

5. Ask patient to sit with hands hanging unsupported. If male, between legs, if female and wearing a dress, hanging over knees. (Observe hands and other body areas.)

6. Ask patient to open mouth. (Observe tongue at rest within mouth.) Do this twice.

7. Ask patient to protrude tongue. (Observe abnormalities of tongue movement.) Do this twice.

***8. Ask patient to tap thumb, with each finger, as rapidly as possible for 10-15 seconds; separately with right hand, then with left hand. (Observe facial and leg movements.)**

9. Flex and extend patient's left and right arms (one at a time). (Note any rigidity and rate on DOTES.)

10. Ask patient to stand up. (Observe in profile. Observe all body areas again, hips included.)

***11. Ask patient to extend both arms outstretched in front with palms down. (Observe trunk, legs, and mouth.)**

***12. Have patient walk a few paces, turn, and walk back to chair. (Observe hands and gait.) Do this twice.**

***Activated movements.**

Reprinted with permission

[1] Available from the Psychopharmacology Research Branch of the National Institute of Mental Health, Washington, DC.

Multi-item rating scales are also available. Simpson, Lee, Zoubek, and Gardos (1979) have developed a 43-item rating scale (and a 17-item abbreviated scale) with the items grouped according to the following areas of the body: face, neck and trunk, and extremities. Additionally, there are categories for rating Parkinsonism-like syndromes and miscellaneous syndromes.

Treatment Strategies

Taylor, Slutnick, and Hoehle (1979) have reported the use of positive and negative feedback combined with overcorrection in successfully reducing the frequency of movements in tardive dyskinesias. Positive and negative feedback involves a short amount of therapy time (10 minutes) in which the patient is informed by the therapist when the movements occur and when they do not occur. Overcorrection, for a period of 10 minutes, involves exaggeration of the particular movement contingent on the initation of the movement.

EMG biofeedback has also been used successfully to treat tardive dyskinesias (Albanese & Gaarder, 1977).

For More Information

Gardos, G., Cole, J., & Brie, R. (1977). The assessment of tardive dyskinesia. *Archives of General Psychiatry, 34*, 1206-1212.

This article reviews the different techniques available for assessing tardive dyskinesia. Included are instrumentation techniques, frequency counts, global ratings, and multi-item rating scales. A discussion of the validity and reliability of the techniques is included. The article can be obtained from George Gardos, M.D., Insitute of Research and Rehabilitation, Boston State Hospital, 591 Morton Street, Boston, MA 02124.

Simpson, G., Lee, J., Zoubok, B., & Gardos, G. (1979). A rating scale for tardive dyskinesia. *Psychopharmacology, 64*, 171-179.

This article contains copies of the 43-item and 17-item rating scales for tardive dyskinesia. All of the categories are objectively defined for both scales, and instructions for administration are included. The article can be obtained from G. M. Simpson, Professor of Psychiatry and Director, USC-MSH Psychopharmacological Services, 11400 Norwalk Blvd., Norwalk, CA 90650.

Taylor, C., Slutnick, S., & Hoehle, W. (1979). The effects of behavioral procedures on tardive dyskinesias. *Behavior Therapy, 10*, 37-45.

This article describes the behavioral treatment of tardive dyskinesia in two case studies. The technique of overcorrection and its components (instructions, feedback, exaggerated rehearsals, and positive and negative reinforcement) are evaluated. The article can be obtained from C. Barr-Taylor, Department of Psychiatry and Behavioral Sciences, Stanford University School of Medicine, Stanford, CA 94305

References

Albanese, H., & Gaarder, K. (1977). Biofeedback treatment of tardive dyskinesia: Two case reports. *American Journal of Psychiatry, 134*, 1149-1150.

Simpson, G., Lee, J., Zoubok, B., & Gardos, G. (1979). A rating scale for tardive dyskinesia. *Psychopharmacology, 64*, 171-179.

Taylor, C., Slutnick, S., & Hoehle, W. (1979). The effects of behavioral procedures on tardive dyskinesias. *Behavior Therapy, 10*, 37-45.

35 Temporomandibular Joint Dysfunction and Pain Syndrome

Assessment Strategies

Temporomandibular joint dysfunction and pain syndrome (TMJDPS) is characterized by pain and tenderness of the muscles of mastication and the temporomandibular joint (TMJ), popping or clicking sounds of the jaw, and limitations of mandibular movements. Other commonly reported symptoms include bruxism, difficulty chewing, and buzzing or ringing in the ear. The patient is likely to complain of pain that is unilateral and described as a dull ache, although it can become sharp and acute. The pain can be located in the back of the head and neck, the jaw, and the area in front of the ear. For many patients, the pain is most intense in the morning.

A dental examination for occlusion, muscle tenderness, and distance of mouth opening width is necessary. A dentist can also rule out other factors that may be causing the problem (e.g., poor fitting dentures or impacted wisdom teeth). Radiographic tests are needed to rule out organic changes in the temporomandibular joint. The popping or clicking sounds of the jaw can be heard with a stethoscope as the patient opens and closes his or her mouth. Behavioral assessment involves a one-to-two week baseline of self-monitoring of jaw pain. Ratings can be made from three times a day to hourly, on a seven-point scale (0 = absence of symptoms, 6 = worst possible severity of symptoms). For patients who experience pain only a few times a day, a behavioral diary can be used. Additional information that can be obtained with continuous recording in a behavioral diary includes: time of day, duration of the pain, who else is present, type of activity engaged in, and any thoughts and feelings. Patients can also estimate the amount of pain-free time per day. An interview with significant others is important to determine if the patient is receiving any reinforcement for pain complaints. The significant other may also supply information regarding any environmental stresses the patient is currently experiencing. An evaluation for depression should also be considered in the initial assessment.

Treatment Strategies

During treatment it is important to continue monitoring all of the patient's symptoms since remission of one symptom is not highly correlated with the remission of other symptoms (Scott & Gregg, 1980).

An attempt should be made to remove any positive reinforcement for pain complaints. Significant others should be instructed to ignore the patient's pain complaints.

Progressive muscle relaxation has been found to be successful for many TMJDPS patients (e.g., Funch & Gale, 1984). It is important that the patient practice the relaxation daily and use the techniques as soon as any muscle tension is evident. Older patients, depressed patients, and patients reinforced for pain benefit least from relaxation techniques (Scott & Gregg, 1980).

A modification of anxiety management training has also been used successfully by Stam, McGrath, & Brooke (1984).

> **Four weekly sessions were developed to enable the client to gain control over her anxiety. As in anxiety management training, each session began with Jacobson's standard progressive relaxation procedure. . . . Then the client was instructed to visualize a relaxing scene with the aid of guided rehearsal. Several detailed descriptions were obtained of actual situations which were relaxing for the client (e.g., lying on a beach on hot summer day). The therapist instructed the client to visualize one of these scenes in each session and, through verbal descriptions of the scene, enable her to vividly re-experience these events. Ordinarily, the visualization of anxiety provoking scenes is included here in an anxiety management training program. This was not done, however, because relaxation itself was anxiety provoking. Successive sessions were aimed at allowing the client to experience control over her anxiety by continuing the progressive relaxation procedure to where she began to feel herself becoming anxious. Instead of panicking, however, she was instructed to return to the point at which the anxiety dissipated. That is, when she became aware of signs of anxiety, such as clenching of the fists or shoulder tightening, she would open her eyes and if necessary, sit up from her reclining position until the anxiety had receded. The therapist would then wait until the client stated that she was free from anxiety before proceeding. The next phase consisted of having her initiate and terminate her anxiety reactions with little or no direct instruction from the therapist. Finally, she was given "homework" to control her anxiety outside the therapy sessions, especially at night prior to falling asleep. [Stam, McGrath, & Brooke, 1984; p. 43]**

If the assessment reveals that an inability to deal with stressful situations is an antecedent to pain, then the use of assertion training, cognitive restructuring, or both may be helpful. Some patients may also need cognitive restructuring to cope with feelings and thoughts about pain. Masseter EMG biofeedback has been generally found to be effective for TMJDPS patients (Carlsson & Gale, 1976; Dohrmann & Laskin, 1978) but may not add to the effectiveness of progressive muscle relaxation alone (Moss, Wedding, & Sanders, 1983).

Funch and Gale (1984) found that younger patients who had experienced TMJ pain for a shorter period of time, who reported bruxing behavior, or who reported more psychosomatic problems benefited more from relaxation therapy than biofeedback. Patients more successful with biofeedback tended to be older, married, and had experienced the TMJ pain for a longer period of time.

For More Information

Moss, R., Garrett, J., & Chiodo, J. (1982). Temporomandibular joint dysfunction and myofacial pain dysfunction syndromes: Parameters, etiology and treatment. *Psychological Bulletin, 92*, 331-346.

This article provides an excellent description of the temporomandibular joint syndrome, the incidence of the disorder, and etiological theories. A short review of behavioral and dental treatment approaches is included. The article can be obtained from Robert Moss, Department of Psychology, University of Mississippi, University, MI 38677.

Reading, A., & Raw, M. (1976). The treatment of mandibular dysfunction pain, possible application of psychological methods. *British Dental Journal, 140*, 201-205.

This article describes the successful use of progressive muscle relaxation with four TMJDPS patients. The article can be obtained from Anthony Reading, Department of Psychiatry, UCLA, Los Angeles, CA 90024.

Scott, D., & Gregg, J. (1980). Myofacial pain of the temporal mandibular joint: A review of the behavioral-relaxation therapies. *Pain, 9*. 231-241.

This article reviews the relaxation and biofeedback treatment studies on TMJDPS. Included is a discussion of the different etiological theories. The article can be obtained from Donald S. Scott, 8036 Timber Lodge, Trail West, Dayton, OH 45459.

Stenn, P., Mothersill, K., & Brook, R. (1979). Biofeedback and a cognitive behavioral approach to treatment of myofacial pain dysfunction syndrome. *Behavior Therapy, 10*, 29-36.

This article describes the successful use of biofeedback combined with a coping skills approach to treat 13 TMJDPS patients. The article can be obtained from P. Stenn, Department of Psychology, University Hospital, P.O. Box 5339, Postal Station A, London, Ontario, Canada N6A 5A5.

References

Carlsson, S., & Gale, E. (1976). Biofeedback treatment for muscle pain associated with the temporomandibular joint. *Journal of Behavior Therapy and Experimental Psychiatry, 7*, 383-385.

Dohrmann, R., & Laskin, D. (1978). An evaluation of electromyographic biofeedback in the treatment of myofacial pain—dysfunction syndrome. *Journal of the American Dental Association, 96*, 656-662.

Funch, D., & Gale, E. (1984). Biofeedback and relaxation therapy for chronic temporomandibular joint pain: Predicting successful outcome. *Journal of Consulting and Clinical Psychology, 52*, 928-935.

Moss, R., Wedding, D., & Sanders, H. (1983). The comparative efficacy of relaxation training and masseter EMG biofeedback in the treatment of TMJ dysfunction. *Journal of Oral Rehabilitation, 10* , 9-17.

Scott, D., & Gregg, J. (1980). Myofacial pain of the temporomandibular joint: A review of the behavioral-relaxation therapies. *Pain, 9*, 231-241.

Stam, H., McGrath, P., & Brook, R. (1984). The treatment of temporomandibular joint syndrome through control of anxiety. *Journal of Behavior Therapy and Experimental Psychiatry, 15*, 41-45.

See Also

Chapter 7. Bruxism
Chapter 30. Pain - Chronic

36 Tics

Assessment Strategies

A tic is an intermittent and recurring muscle spasm. Before any behavioral treatment is initiated, a medical or neurological exam, or both, should be completed to rule out any organic cause of the tic, such as a spasm, chorea, or tremor. Some of the important differences between an organically caused tic and a psychogenic tic are: 1) the psychogenic tic is under voluntary control, 2) reflexes are unimpaired in the psychogenic tic, 3) the execution of the psychogenic tic often reduces tension, and 4) if the tic occurs during sleep, it is likely to be of organic origin.

The minimal behavioral assessment should involve a frequency count. Because these behaviors tend to occur at a very high frequency, a wrist counter is recommended. In addition to frequency, a behavioral analysis diary should be used to determine any antecedents or consequences maintaining the behavior. One common antecedent tends to be anxiety-provoking situations. Frequency counts can be validated by having an outside observer, frequently a significant other, do unobtrusive time-sampling.

Some other useful measures are the patient's rating of the intensity of the tic and the percent of a day during which he or she experiences the tic. Therapist observations in session, which can also be videotaped, can serve as another assessment of frequency.

Treatment Strategies

The initial treatment can be a continuation of the self-monitoring. Daily totals can be graphed by the patient and reported to the therapist by phone. The phone call to the therapist can be used to provide opportunities to reinforce lowered frequencies. To use this technique, the baseline count of the tic should not be too high, for then the recording would disrupt the patient's normal daily activities. If the self-monitoring is effective in reducing tics, it can be faded out gradually.

If the simple self-monitoring treatment is not successful, the use of habit-reversal should be attempted. Miltenberger, Fuqua, and McKinley (1985) describe the components of the procedure as applied to tics as follows:

> **1. *Awareness training:* Subjects engaged in response description and detection procedures in which they described their tics while watching a portion of their videotape, identified instances of the tic occurring on the videotape, and identified actual instances of the tic occurring in session. Subjects practiced until they could reliably detect occurrences of their tic.**
>
> **2. *Situations and habit inconvenience review:* Subjects reviewed all situations in which the tics occurred. Subjects also listed all the inconveniences and embarrassments resulting from the occurrence of their tics. The list was reviewed in session and subjects were instructed to review the list daily.**
>
> **3. *Relaxation:* Subjects were instructed in a deep breathing form of relaxation while**

in a sitting position. Subjects were instructed to practice the relaxation at least once per day for 10 min.

4. *Competing response:* Subjects learned a competing response . . . selected to be incompatible with their particular tic. They practiced the competing response for 3 min contingent on each occurrence of the tic for the remainder of the session. They were instructed to engage in the competing response for 3 min contingent on the occurrence of each tic and to practice the competing response for 15 min each day.

5. *Social support:* Each subject was instructed to have a significant other (i.e., spouse, friend, child) praise him/her for not engaging in the tic and to prompt the subject to "do your exercise" when caught engaging in the tic. Subjects were also instructed to seek previously avoided situations once the tic decreased in frequency. [p. 44]

Miltenberger et al. (1985) also found that just using the awareness training and competing response components was as effective as the entire habit-reversal technique. Azrin, Nunn, and Frantz (1980; see Table 36-1) describe the competing responses used for seven different tics.

Table 36-1

DESCRIPTION OF THE COMPETING REACTION FOR VARIOUS TICS

Tic	*Competing Reaction*
Backwards	With the head in a centered position, contract head jerking neck flexors so that head tilts slightly downward. Neck appears shortened and bulged. (If this reaction is inadequate, push the chin into the sternum. Gradually decrease the contraction so that the head is raised off the sternum in the more natural head-upright position.)
Sideways	Keep head in center position and contract neck head jerking flexors so that head tilts slightly downward. (If this reaction cannot be maintained for 3 minutes, or is inadequate, put hand on side of face and push the head in the direction opposite to the tic.) After strengthening of opposing neck muscles, change to the isometric neck flexor reaction without the hand assist.
Shoulder jerking	Contract shoulders by depressing the shoulders as far as they will go while keeping the arms close to the body.
Head shaking	Shift head posture from very erect or angled to drooping or tilting the head slightly forward. Slightly contract neck muscles that oppose shaking movements.
Wrist tics	Push hands on arms of chairs, desk, leg, etc. and contract the muscles so that hands are pushing opposite the tic movement (i.e., contract hands down if the wrist jerks upward).
Neck stretching	Contract neck flexors and depress head so that neck appears shortened.
Moving shoulder	Contract shoulder by depressing the shoulder arm as if downward and pressing arm to side of body, disengaging sleeve from jacket

[Azrin et al., 1980; p. 174]

All other aspects of the general habit-reversal technique, including awareness training, habit control motivation, and generalization training are included in the treatment of tics.

Negative, or massed, practice has been used successfully with some patients. The muscle movements involved should as accurately as possible match the involuntary tic. The massed practice should be done in front of a mirror. Videotaping the tic prior to the massed practice and showing the tape to the patient may help the patient to accurately reproduce the tic. The use of a metronome as a cue may facilitate the massed practice. The addition of the thought "this is what I'm not supposed to do" during the massed practice may be beneficial. Also, the use of aversive olfactory substances, contingent on each evocation of the tic, may add to the effectiveness of this technique (Knepler & Sewall, 1974). The frequency of massed practice in each session has not been standardized. As little as five one-minute trials with one-minute rests between trials and as much as six hours of continuous practice followed by several weeks rest have been used successfully. Patients should report feeling fatigued at the end of each practice session.

If short massed practice sessions are used, practice can continue at home for ten-minute periods about six times per day. The patient should maintain the self-monitoring throughout treatment. For generalization purposes the therapy sessions can gradually introduce more people into the room. These observers can initially be silent, but eventually create some anxiety by being critical of the patient. At the conclusion of treatment the patient should be encouraged to cut the practice sessions down to about 30-second periods once per hour. Full practice should be resumed if relapse occurs. Playing the initial videotape of the patient's tic near the conclusion of treatment may serve as an added reinforcement.

Patients who are prone to develop anxiety may not be suitable for massed practice. This type of patient may have difficulty reproducing the tic, or the use of massed practice may actually increase the tic if the anxiety is not treated. Tics are often related to anxiety in social situations. The use of progressive muscle relaxation may be a helpful adjunct for many patients with tics, but may not be effective by itself (St. James-Roberts & Powell, 1979).

O'Brien and Brennan (1979) have successfully combined relaxation training, habit reversal, desensitization, and the use of a prosthetic response prevention device to successfully treat a patient with severe facial tic. They describe the use of the response prevention device as follows:

> **. . . the client indicated that the movement of the jaw outward might serve as a conditioned stimulus for eliciting anxiety. Therfore, a physical restraint device consisting of velbrow straps and a hockey chin cup was used to control the onset of this stimulus. The straps were extended from the chin cup over the top of the client's head and behind the neck. They could be tightened to restrict excessive jaw movement. The device also provided the client with more feedback about the onset of the jaw movements. . . . Sessions, at this point, included the client wearing her chin strap, relaxing, and visualizing graded scenes of events associated with anxiety. [p. 260]**

It is also important to deal with any social reinforcement or secondary gain provided by the symptom. It may be necessary to have significant others put the attention paid to the tics on extinction and positively reinforce reduced rates of tic behavior. Barrett (1962) achieved some success with an operant technique. However, this procedure involves the use of elaborate equipment.

For More Information

Azrin, N., & Nunn, R. (1973). Habit-reversal: A method of eliminating nervous habits and tics. *Behavior Research and Therapy, 11*, 619-628.

This article contains an excellent description of the habit-reversal technique, including suggestions of different competing responses. The article can be obtained from N. Azrin, Nova University, Psychology Department, 3301 College Ave., Fort Lauderdale, FL 33314.

Hersen, M., & Eisler, R. (1973). Behavioral approaches to study and treatment of psychogenic tics. *Genetic Psychology Monographs, 87*, 289-312.

This article is an excellent review of the definition of tics, the genesis and reinforcement of tics, and different behavioral treatment approaches. Two case studies are included. The article can be obtained from Michael Hersen, Western Psychiatric Institute and Clinic, Department of Psychiatry, 3811 O'Hara St., Pittsburgh, PA, 15213.

Nicassio, F., Liberman, R., Patterson, R., and Ramirez, E. (1972). The treatment of tics by negative practice. *Journal of Behavior Therapy and Experimental Psychiatry, 3*, 281-287.

This article describes the use of negative practice with two patients. Only one case was successfully treated. The article can be obtained from Frank Nicassio, 511 N.W. 8th St., Pendleton, OR 97801.

References

Azrin, N., Nunn, R., & Frantz, S. (1980). Habit-reversal versus negative practice treatment of nervous tics. *Behavior Therapy, 11*, 169-178.

Barrett, B. (1962). Reduction in rate of multiple tics by free operant conditioning methods. *Journal of Nervous and Mental Disease, 15*, 187-195.

Knepler, K., & Sewall, S. (1974). Negative practice paired with smelling salts in the treatment of a tic. *Journal of Behavior Therapy and Experimental Psychiatry, 5*, 189-192.

Miltenberger, R., Fuqua, R., & McKinley, T. (1985). Habit reversal with muscle tics: Replication and component analysis. *Behavior Therapy, 16*, 39-50.

O'Brien, J., & Brennan, J. (1979). The elimination of a severe long term facial tic and vocal distortion with multi-facet behavior therapy. *Journal of Behavior Therapy and Experimental Psychiatry, 10*, 257-261.

St. James-Roberts, N., & Powell, G. (1979). A case-study comparing the effects of relaxation and massed practice upon tic frequency. *Behavior Research and Therapy, 17*, 401-403.

See Also

Chapter 5. Blepharospasm

37 Tinnitus

Assessment Strategies

Tinnitus aurium is defined as a ringing sound subjectively identified as being within the ear. Tinnitus cerebri is the term which refers to a ringing sound subjectively localized within the head (Grossan, 1976). Tinnitus may be further classified as either subjective, in which it is audible only to the patient, or objective, in which it is also audible to an observer (Marlowe, 1973).

Marlowe (1973) offers the following description of tinnitus:

> **Patient descriptions of tinnitus are quite varied but often mentioned are a "buzzing," a "ringing," or a "sound of escaping steam" noise. This may be present intermittently or constantly, and if intermittent, may be rhythmic in character and noted by the patient to be synchronous with his pulse. Tinnitus with this characteristic is most likely of vascular origin. Some patients may complain of a grating sound or an intermittent clicking, which is repetitive but not rhythmic. This may be due to a condition of involuntary contraction of the muscles of mastication, so-called "tensor tympani clonus."**
>
> **The intensity of tinnitus, as reported by different patients varies considerably. In some, the noise is audible only under conditions of extreme quiet, while in others it is so loud that at no time are they free from the distressing sound. [pp. 162-163]**

Assessment of tinnitus is complicated by the clinician's reliance on the patient's subjective description. A neuro-otologic and audiologic evaluation should be conducted. In assessing severity of tinnitus, two variables are commonly measured: pitch and volume. Psychoacoustic ratings of pitch and volume may be obtained.

Subjective ratings of tinnitus severity may also be obtained. Borton, Moore and Clark (1981) employed a 10-segment scale. They describe the scale as follows:

> **Each scale was partially anchored along its continuum using descriptors provided by the subject. For example, on the tinnitus severity scale a rating of zero indicated that tinnitus was absent, while a rating of 10 characterized it as a "loud piercing tone." [p. 40]**

Patients can also rate the annoyance created by the tinnitus on a seven-point Likert scale (1 denotes no annoyance, and 7 the most annoying the tinnitus has ever been). Ireland, Wilson, Tonkin, and Platt-Hepworth (1985) included a more comprehensive subjective evaluation of tinnitus, where the patient was asked to make the following ratings:

> **(1) number of times tinnitus occurred; (2) percentage of the time during which Ss were aware of their tinnitus; (3) rated loudness of tinnitus (0-4 point scale). Ss were instructed to make these ratings at the end of each day throughout each monitoring period. [p. 425]**

Associated somatic complaints, including sleep disturbance, may also be assessed.

Hallam and Jakes (1985) assessed the degree to which tinnitus interfered with activity level. They describe the assessment as follows: "Disability was measured by a 23-item checklist of daily activities (DQ) which were rated for interference by tinnitus (i.e. 'not at all,' 'a little,' 'a lot,' 'no opportunity')" (p. 692).

Borton et al. (1981) obtained subjective ratings of annoyance with tinnitus via a 10-segment scale described as follows: "A rating of zero on the annoyance scale was used if tinnitus was absent (therefore, not annoying), while a rating of 10 indicated that the subject found her tinnitus 'extremely annoying'" (p. 40).

The clinician may also wish to assess the patient's beliefs, attitudes, and expectations associated with tinnitus. Hallam and Jakes (1985) have developed a 40-item questionnaire, the Tinnitus Effects Questionnaire (TEQ), which can be used for this purpose.

Finally, for many patients complaining of tinnitus, depression and anxiety may also need to be assessed.

Treatment Strategies

Relaxation training has had mixed results in the treatment of tinnitus. Jakes, Hallam, Rachman and Hinchcliffe (1986) found that five sessions of progressive muscle relaxation were effective in reducing the annoyance caused by the tinnitus and in reducing the interference the tinnitus caused with daily activities. However, progressive muscle relaxation was not effective in reducing the loudness nor the intrusiveness of the tinnitus. They also found no advantage in adding a distraction technique (i.e., attention-switching) to the relaxation training.

Ireland, Wilson, Tonkin, and Platt-Hepworth (1985) employed a progressive relaxation procedure with a group of tinnitus patients. Relaxation was not successful in reducing subjective tinnitus or associated somatic complaints. Grossan (1976) successfully used frontalis EMG biofeedback with a group of tinnitus patients.

For More Information

Grossan, M. (1976). Treatment of subjective tinnitus with biofeedback. *Ear, Nose, and Throat Journal, 55*, 314-318.

This article describes a biofeedback treatment procedure with a group of tinnitus patients. It provides information on the assessment of tinnitus and a detailed outline of the intervention. The article can be obtained from S. Jakes, Institute of Laryngology and Otology, 330-332 Gray's Inn Road, London WC1X 8EE, England.

Jakes, S., Hallam, R., Rachman, S., & Hinchcliffe, R. (1986). The effects of reassurance, relaxation training and distraction on chronic tinnitus sufferers. *Behavior Research and Therapy, 24*, 497-507.

This article describes a group study using progressive relaxation training and distraction techniques to treat tinnitus. An excellent description of the assessment methods are included. The article can be obtained from S. Jakes, Institute of Laryngology and Otology, 330-332 Gray's Inn Road, London WC1X 8EE, England.

References

Borton, T., Moore, W., & Clark, S. (1981). Electromyographic feedback treatment for tinnitus aurium. *Journal of Speech and Hearing Disorders, 46*, 39-45.

Elfner, L., May, J., Moore, J., & Mendelson, J. (1981). Effects of EMG and thermal feedback training on tinnitus: A case study. *Biofeedback and Self-Regulation, 6*, 517-521.

Grossan, M. (1976). Treatment of subjective tinnitus with biofeedback. *Ear, Nose, and Throat Journal, 55*, 314-318.

Hallam, R., & Jakes, S. (1985). Case histories and shorter communications. *Behavior Research and Therapy, 23*, 691-694.

House, J. (1978). Treatment of severe tinnitus with biofeedback training. *Laryngoscope, 88*, 406-412.

Ireland, C., Wilson, P., Tonkin, J., & Platt-Hepworth, S. (1985). An evaluation of relaxation training in the treatment of tinnitus. *Behavior Research and Therapy, 23*, 423-430.

Jakes, S., Hallam, R., Rachman, S., & Hinchcliffe, R. (1986). The effects of reassurance, relaxation training and distraction on chronic tinnitus sufferers. *Behavior Research and Therapy, 24*, 497-507.

Marlowe, F. (1973). Effective treatment of tinnitus through hypnotherapy. *American Journal of Clinical Hypnosis, 15*, 162-165.

38 Tourette's Syndrome

Assessment Strategies

Gilles de la Tourette's is a syndrome of multiple tics, "compulsive jerking of involuntary musculature in the face, neck, or extremities, combined with coprolalia, echolalia, or of other spasmodic involuntary noises" (Thomas, Abrams, & Johnson, 1971; p. 159). A thorough neurological and medical exam should precede any behavioral assessment.

The first step in a behavioral assessment is to identify the components (e.g., separate tics) of the syndrome. Following this identification, the frequency of the tics should be recorded. In many patients the presence of multiple tics may necessitate choosing two or three major tics to monitor at first. Because of the high frequency of occurrence of these tics, a time sampling procedure is recommended. When patients record their time-sampled tic frequency they should also note their general situation at the time of the occurrence of the tics. This is important to determine if there are any specific stimulus conditions that effect tic frequency. The therapist can supplement these recordings by taking the patient into real-life situations that he or she might normally avoid, and monitor the frequency of the tics in these situations.

Other assessment strategies used for tics can also be used for Tourette's syndrome.

Treatment Strategies

For many patients, self-monitoring alone may be successful in reducing the frequency of each tic. The effectiveness of this technique can best be determined by applying a multiple baseline design to the different tics involved in the syndrome.

If self-monitoring does not reduce the frequency of the behavior to an acceptable level, relaxation training and systematic desensitization can be added (e.g., Thomas, Abrams, & Johnson, 1971). After learning the relaxation skills, the patient can be instructed to use relaxation following occurrence of the behavior. Muscular relaxation is incompatible with many of the tic behaviors. Systematic desensitization can involve scenes that would normally produce muscle tension. These scenes can be generated from the patient's self-report and observations by the therapist. The hierarchy could start with situations that normally produce little or no muscular tension. In vivo exposure can supplement any imaginal exposure.

Cue-controlled relaxation alone has not been found to be effective in reducing the tic frequency in Tourette's patients (Turpin & Powell, 1984). Massed practice has generally been ineffective in treating Tourette's syndrome (Nicassio, Lieberman, Patterson, & Ramirez, 1972; Hollandsworth & Bausinger, 1978). Hollandsworth and Bausinger (1978) found that massed practice actually increased the occurrence of coprolalic responses in one patient. Clark (1966) used massed practice to successfully reduce the coprolalic responses of two patients.

> **A massed practice regimen was set up in which the patient was asked to repeat the currently most frequent obscenity as often as possible (and as loudly as was feasible in the treatment setting) until he/she could no longer succeed in saying it even once every minute. The number of repetitions was recorded on a unit counter by the therapist who noted the total at 30 second intervals until it remained the same for 60 seconds. [Clark, 1966; p. 773]**

Massed practice is usually carried out on a daily basis until the patient becomes fatigued. It may also be possible to apply the habit reversal technique used with tics to the Tourette's syndrome.

For More Information

Thomas, E., Abrams, K., & Johnson, J. (1971). Self-monitoring and reciprocal inhibition in the modification of multiple tics of Gilles de la Tourette's syndrome. *Journal of Behavior Therapy and Experimental Psychiatry, 2*, 159-171.

This article details the use of self-monitoring and systematic desensitization in treating an inpatient case of Tourette's syndrome. An excellent description of assessment procedures is included. The article can be obtained from Edwin Thomas, University of Michigan School of Social Work, 1065 Frieze Building, Ann Arbor, MI 48104.

References

Clark, D. (1966). Behavior therapy of Gilles da la Tourette's syndrome. *British Journal of Psychiatry, 112*, 771-778.

Hollandsworth, J., Jr., & Vausinger, L. (1978). Unsuccessful use of massed practice in the treatment of Gilles de la Tourette's syndrome. *Psychological Reports, 43*, 671-677.

Nicassio, F., Lieberman, R., Patterson, R., & Ramirez, E. (1972). Treatment of tics by negative practice. *Journal of Behavioral Therapy and Experimental Psychiatry, 3*, 281-287.

Thomas, E., Abrams, K., & Johnson, J. (1971). Self-monitoring and reciprocal inhibition in the modification of multiple tics of Gilles de la Tourette's syndrome. *Journal of Behavioral Therapy and Experimental Psychiatry, 2*, 159-171.

Turpin, G., & Powell, G. (1984). Effects of massed practice and cue-controlled relaxation on tic frequency in Gilles de la Tourette's Syndrome. *Behavior Research and Therapy, 22*, 165-178.

See Also

Chapter 36. Tics

39 Type A Behavior

Assessment Strategies

Type A behavior is a pattern characterized by a highly competitive, achievement- and recognition-oriented attitude. The type A individual tends to be fast moving, impatient, and feels pressured for time. Type A individuals tend to have a hard time relaxing but are very physically and mentally alert and quick. They may also react to frustration with anger. Type A individuals are at increased risk for coronary heart disease. There are two excellent measures for assessing the presence of type A behavior. The Jenkins Activity Survey[1] (Jenkins, Rosenman, and Zizanski, 1972) is a self-report questionnaire that measures type A behavior and yields three factor scores: speed and impatience, job involvement, and hard-driving and competitive.

A structured oral interview has been developed by Rosenman et al. (1964). During this 15- to 20-minute interview, ratings of the degree of type A behavior are based on the content of responses, motor behaviors, voice and facial qualities, emotional responses, and spontaneous comments. A patient needs to exhibit one or more psychomotor manifestations or react positively to one or more of the direct behavioral tests to be considered a type A personality. Friedman (1979) indicates that most patients will display about half of the indicators of each of the categories during the interview. Friedman, Thoresen, and Gill (1981) have also developed a videotaped structured interview.

Two quick self-rating scales are available. Bortner (1969) developed a 14-item scale, and Haynes, Feinleiv, Levine, Scotch, and Kannel (1978) have developed a 10-item scale called the Framingham Questionnaire (see Table 39-1).

Herman, Blumenthal, Black, and Chesney (1981) have developed a 65-item adjective checklist that aids in identifying the type A individual. Specific type A behaviors can also be assessed. Examples of specific behaviors include: anger, number of hours and overtime hours worked, number of recreation hours, number of vacation days, weight, and number of cigarettes smoked. Additionally, the physiological measures of serum cholesterol, blood pressure, and serum triglycerides can be assessed. However, many programs that are successful in changing the general type A behavior pattern may have no effect on these physiological variables.

Treatment Strategies

The most frequent treatment for type A behavior is some form of anxiety management. To obtain compliance, it may be helpful to explain to patients that their efficiency and performance may increase if they learn to control stress. Relaxation training with daily home practice is included in all of the anxiety

[1] Available from the Psychological Corporation, 757 Third Avenue, New York, NY 10017.

Table 39-1

FRAMINGHAM QUESTIONNAIRE

Name ________________________________
Date ___________________
Age ___ Sex ___

Are you currently: __ employed __ retired __ unemployed __ housewife
(check one)

If employed, please indicate occupation: ________________________________

Below is a list of several traits or qualities that describe people. For each one, please mark a check "✓ " in the box that applies to you. Since there are no right or wrong answers, we are mainly interested in the answers that describe you the best.

Describes me:

	Very well	*Fairly well*	*Somewhat*	*Not at all*
1. Having a strong need to excel (be the best) in most things	❒	❒	❒	❒
2. Usually pressed for time	❒	❒	❒	❒
3. Being hard-driving and competitive	❒	❒	❒	❒
4. Being bossy or dominating	❒	❒	❒	❒
5. Eating too quickly	❒	❒	❒	❒

Now we would like to know how you have generally felt during an average day in your regular line of work. If retired or unemployed, please refer to your last job. If a housewife, please refer to your housework.

	Yes	*No*
6. Have you often felt pressed for time?	❒	❒
7. Has your work often stayed with you so that you were thinking about it after working hours?	❒	❒
8. Has your work often stretched you to the very limits of your energy and capacity?	❒	❒
9. Have you often felt uncertain, uncomfortable or dissatisfied with how well you were doing your work?	❒	❒
10. Do you get quite upset when you have to wait for anything?	❒	❒

management programs. Daily monitoring of tension levels and situations associated with increases and decreases of tension can easily be incorporated in any type of behavioral intervention program. Cue-related relaxation can then be paired with stressful situations; for example, relaxation every time the patient enters a crowded highway. Cardiac stress management training (Suinn, 1975) combines anxiety management training and visuomotor behavioral rehearsal. Suinn and Bloom (1975) describe the procedure as follows:

> **In the first stage subjects are taught deep muscle relaxation. In the second stage anxiety is aroused through imagery and subjects are trained to identify the particular muscular or physiological cues accompanying anxiety arousal. In the third stage subjects gain practice in learning to recognize these cues and to engage in relaxation as a coping response. In visuomotor behavior rehearsal, subjects utilize imagery to rehearse alternative behaviors to type A behaviors, prior to trying these out in vivo. [p. 27]**

This type of program can be completed in three to eight weeks with two to three sessions per week, and can be conducted in groups. Anxiety management training has also been successfully used in dealing with just the anger/hostility component of type A behavior (Hart, 1984). After learning deep muscle relaxation, patients were deliberately stressed by using anger or hostility imagery. The patients were to observe where and how stress was experienced. The patients eventually were taught to use relaxation to cope with the stress.

Self-control training has also been used as one component in a comprehensive behavior therapy program for reducing type A behaviors (Levenkron, Cohen, Mueller, & Fisher, 1983). Subjects were taught to anticipate situations in which they responded with type A behaviors and to generate personal self-control strategies. Examples include: "Removing one's wristwatch when unavoidably delayed, taking less work home in the evening, adjusting personal schedules, and choosing alternative routes to work" (Levenkron, Cohen, Mueller, & Fisher, 1983; p. 194). Any strategy used should be appropriate for the individual's lifestyle. A program of self-rewards and self-punishments can also be set up to maintain new behaviors.

Cognitive-behavioral techniques have also been found to be successful in modifying type A behavior. Jenni and Wollersheim (1979) used rational emotive therapy and had patients rehearse in imagination real-life situations associated with the type A behavior pattern, such as time pressure or competitiveness. Thurman (1985a, 1985b) successfully used cognitive behavior modification in eight two-hour group sessions focusing on changing maladaptive beliefs related to anger, hostility, competitive drive, and impatience in the type A personality. Homework assignments were used to help the individual develop non-type A responses to typical daily problem situations (e.g., waiting in line or traffic). There was no advantage in adding assertion training to the cognitive behavior modification techniques. Additionally, some individuals were resistant to the homework assignments because of added time pressure.

Cognitive therapy techniques can also be added to a stress management program. Changing self-statements related to type A situations may be helpful.

Direct modification of specific behavioral changes may also be useful for some type A patients. Examples include: decreasing involvement in or resigning from committees or organizations, delegating responsibilities, walking and talking at a slower pace, and learning better time management skills.

It may be more difficult to intervene with patients who have not had a myocardial infarction. For these patients it is important to reassure them that the treatment program will not attempt to modify their level of achievement. To increase motivation in patients who have recently suffered a myocardial infarction, it is advisable to make contact while the patient is still in the hospital.

Exercise programs and diet modification may be useful components to a comprehensive treatment program to reduce type A behaviors.

For More Information

Friedman, M., & Rosenman, R. (1974). *Type A behavior and your heart.* New York: Fawcett.

This is a self-help book that is appropriate for patient use. The book describes the type A pattern and methods to modify the pattern. The book can be obtained from Fawcett Books Publishing Company, 201 East 50th St., New York, NY 10022.

Hersen, M., & Bellack, A. (1986). Coronary-prone behavior patterns. In M. Hersen & A. Bellack (Eds.) *Handbook of clinical behavior therapy with adults* (pp. 400-409). New York: Plenum.

This chapter emphasizes the pratical application of the different assessment and treatment strategies. Included is a good discussion of patient motivation and a partial transcript of an interview with a type A behavior patient. The book can be obtained from Plenum Publishing Corporation, 233 Spring Street, New York, NY 10003.

Jenni, M., & Wollersheim, J. (1979). Cognitive therapy, stress management training, and the type A behavior pattern. *Cognitive Therapy and Research, 3*, 61-73.

This article compares the use of Ellis's cognitive therapy to Suinn's stress management training in modifying type A behavior in a group study. The article can be obtained from Mary Jenni, Life Development Center, 1207 Mount Ave., Missoula, MT 59801.

Levenkron, J., Cohen, J., Mueller, H., & Fisher, E. (1983). Modifying the type A coronary-prone behavior pattern. *Journal of Consulting and Clinical Psychology, 51*, 192-204.

This article briefly reviews the previous studies that have attempted to modify type A behavior. A comprehensive behavior therapy program emphasizing relaxation, stress management, and self-control is compared to group support and brief information treatments. Included is a good description of different assessment techniques. The article can be obtained from Jeffrey Levenkron, Division of Behavioral and Psychosocial Medicine, Department of Psychiatry, University of Rochester Medical Center, 300 Crittenden Blvd., Rochester, NY 14642.

Suinn, R. (1982). Intervention in type A behavior. *Journal of Consulting and Clinical Psychology, 50*, 933-949.

This comprehensive review describes the various assessment instruments and physiological correlates of type A behavior. Intervention studies with healthy individuals and individuals with cardiovascular disease are then reviewed. Physiological and stress changes are discussed and a thorough evaluation of the methodology issues of the reported research is provided. The article can be obtained from Richard Suinn, Psychology Department, Colorado State University, Fort Collins, CO 80523.

References

Bortner, R. (1969). A short rating scale as a potential measure of pattern A behavior. *Journal of Chronic Diseases, 22*, 87-91.

Friedman, M. (1979). The modification of type A behavior in post-infarction patients. *American Heart Journal, 97*, 551-560.

Friedman, M., Thoreson, C., & Gill, J. (1981). Type A behavior: Its possible role, detection and alteration in patients with ischemic heart disease. In J. Hurst (Ed.), *Update V: The heart*. New York: McGraw-Hill.

Hart, K. (1980). *Stress management training for type A individuals*. Unpublished manuscript.

Haynes, S., Feinleiv, N., Levine, S., Scotch, N., & Kannel, W. (1978). The relationship of psychosocial factors to coronary heart disease in the Framingham study: Prevalence of coronary heart disease. *American Journal of Epidemiology, 107*, 384-402.

Herman, S., Blumenthal, J., Block, G., & Chesney, N. (1981). Self-ratings of type A (coronary prone) adults: Do type A's know they are type A's? *Psychosomatic Medicine, 43*, 405-413.

Jenkins, C., Rosenman, R., & Zizanski, S. (1972). The Jenkins Activity Survey for Health Prediction, form b. Boston: Published by the authors.

Jenni, M., & Wollersheim, J. (1979). Cognitive therapy, stress management training, and the type A behavior pattern. *Cognitive Therapy and Research, 3*, 61-73.

Levenkron, J., Cohen, J., Mueller, H., & Fisher, E. (1983). Modifying the type A coronary-prone behavior pattern. *Journal of Consulting and Clinical Psychology, 32*, 192-204.

Rosenman, R., Friedman, M., Straus, R., Wurm, M., Kositchek, R., Hahn, W., & Werthessen, N. (1964). A predictive study of coronary heart disease.

Journal of the American Medical Association, 189, 15-22.

Suinn, R. (1975). The cardiac stress management program for type A patients. *Cardiac Rehabilitation, 5*, 13-16.

Suinn, R., & Bloom, L. (1978). Anxiety management training for pattern A behavior. *Journal of Behavioral Medicine, 1*, 25-35.

Thurman, C. (1985a). Effectiveness of cognitive-behavioral treatments in reducing type A behavior among university faculty. *Journal of Counseling Psychology, 32*, 74-83.

Thurman, C. (1985b). Effectiveness of cognitive-behavioral treatments in reducing type A behavior among university faculty - one year later. *Journal of Counseling Psychology, 32*, 445-448.

40 Ulcers

Assessment Strategies

A peptic ulcer is a lesion in the wall of the gastrointestinal tract caused by an excess secretion of hydrochloric acid and pepsin. The most frequently reported symptom is pain in the upper abdomen. Initial diagnosis should be made by a physician who may obtain x-ray confirmation of the ulcer. Behavioral assessment can focus on the amount of antacid (or other prescribed medication) consumed per day and a daily rating of severity of ulcer-related pain on a 1-to-5 scale (1 denotes no pain all day, 3 pain during the day relieved by antacid, and 5 pain during the day which is not relieved by antacid and which causes a disruption of planned activities).

Additionally, the patient should be administered general measures of anxiety (e.g., State-Trait Anxiety Inventory) and assertiveness (e.g., Rathus Assertiveness Inventory).

Treatment Strategies

Medication and pain records should be continued throughout treatment to monitor the effects of the interventions.

Anxiety, unassertiveness, or both are likely to be significant factors in a majority of ulcer patients. A combination of anxiety management training and assertiveness training has been found very effective and long lasting in relieving ulcer symptomatology (Brooks & Richardson, 1980). Cognitive restructuring was included in their anxiety and assertiveness treatments. Relaxation training can also be included. In addition, flooding has been used to reduce the anxiety of the patient with ulcers (Stambaugh, 1977).

There have been mixed results in using frontalis EMG biofeedback in treating ulcers. Beaty (1976) successfully treated ulcer patients with a combination of frontalis EMG biofeedback and relaxation training. However, Aleo and Nicassio (1978) found no benefit from these procedures until cognitive restructuring and imagery were added.

For More Information

Brooks, G., & Richardson, F. (1980). Emotional skills training: A treatment program for duodenal ulcer. *Behavior Therapy, 11*, 198-207.

This article describes the use of anxiety management training and assertion training in a group study of duodenal ulcer patients. Included is a good description of assessment methods and examples of the application of the techniques used for typical patient complaints. The article can be obtained from Gary Brooks, Psychology Service, Olin E. Teague Veterans Center, Temple, TX 76501.

References

Aleo, S., & Nicassio, P. (1978). Auto-regulation of duodenal ulcer disease: A preliminary report of four cases. *Proceedings of the Biofeedback Society of America* (pp. 278-281). Denver, CO.

Beaty, E. (1976). Feedback assisted relaxation training as a treatment for peptic ulcers. *Biofeedback and Self-Regulation, 1*, 323-324.

Brooks, G., & Richardson, F. (1980). Emotional skills training: A treatment program for duodenal ulcer. *Behavior Therapy, 11*, 198-207.

Stambaugh, E. (1977). Audio-taped flooding in outpatient treatment of somatic complaints. *Journal of Behavior Therapy and Experimental Psychiatry, 8*, 173-176.

41 Urination — Excessive

Assessment Strategies

Excessive urination can refer to an increase in the frequency of urination (pollakiuria) or the passage of an unusually large volume of urine (polyuria), or both. Urinary frequency of more than eight to ten times per day or more than once nocturnally, or both, is considered to be excessive for individuals in the 18-to-25 age range (Yates & Poole, 1972).

A physical exam is needed to determine if the urinary problem has an organic cause. Excessive urination can result from diabetes, genitourinary infections, side effects from medications, tumors, stones, and other physical disorders. Neurogenic (spastic) bladder is a condition that results in decreased control of bladder functions. A cystomogram can be used to determine if there are any physiological abnormalities of the bladder and the volume of the bladder when the patient experiences the urge to urinate. Behavioral assessment of excessive urination should focus on the urge to urinate, the frequency of urination, and the amount of urination. For the first one to three weeks the patient should monitor both frequency and urges. Additionally, the volume of urine should be measured at random times during the baseline. The patient can be given a graduated urinal to aid in this recording. It is also important to record activity that was occurring prior to the urination or the urge to urinate. These activities should be rated for amount of anxiety by using a SUDS level. An example of a behavioral assessment form for excessive urination is shown in Figure 41-1.

Alternative behavioral assessment involves having the patient drink successive 10 ml samples of fluid without urinating. After each 10 ml sample, the patient can rate his or her urge to urinate on a 1 to 10 scale. It also may be important to have the patient rate the degree of change in freedom of activity, since many patients avoid situations because of the fear of urinating. Cohen and Reed (1968) suggest the following scale: "Symptom-free—no restriction of activity (+3), much increased freedom of activity (+2), slightly increased freedom of activity (+1), no change (0), or decreased freedom of activity (-1)" (p. 1277).

Treatment Strategies

The patient should continue to keep a record of urinary urges and frequency during treatment. Based on the assessment, the patient may require one or more of the techniques described to treat the disorder.

If the assessment reveals a pattern of anxiety-arousing situations, or simply high anxiety ratings associated with urination, then an anxiety reduction procedure should be initiated. Relaxation training and systematic desensitization have been used successfully with excessive urination (Cohen & Reed, 1968; Rovetto, 1983). In addition to a hierarchy of the situations that elicit the anxiety, some patients will need a second hierarchy of the symptoms themselves, if these symptoms generate additional anxiety. To promote generalization, in vivo desensiti-

Date Time	Urge (g) Urination (u)	Behavior prior to urination	SUDS	Volume of urine (every 5th time)

Figure 41-1
Behavioral Analysis for Urination

zation can follow imaginal desensitization.

Urinary scheduling is effective in increasing the latency between voiding. Based on the patient's baseline data, a urinary schedule can be constructed. For example, if the mean interval between urinations during baseline is 50 minutes, the initial treatment schedule could begin with one-hour intervals. For some patients it may be necessary to start the schedule with the actual time interval obtained during the baseline period. Patients are encouraged to keep to the schedule even if there is no urge to urinate at the scheduled time. When the patient is easily able to maintain the time interval, it can be extended by five to ten minutes. Patients can be taught relaxation training and utilize the relaxation exercises when the urge to urinate becomes physically uncomfortable.

Between urination intervals patients can be encouraged to engage in behaviors incompatible with the opportunity to urinate. Examples include taking walks or going shopping at a place where toilet facilities are not readily available. A self-reward program can be set up to reinforce successes in keeping to the schedule. Additionally, a response cost can occur for each failure to maintain the schedule. Masur (1976) suggests that for each minute the patient deviates from the schedule, three minutes of additional bathroom time can be used as a fine. During this time the patient cannot engage in any other activity (e.g., smoking or reading).

Urinary scheduling may even be effective for some cases of neurogenic bladder disorder (O'Neill, 1982). However, the ultimate goal of the program may have to be considerably shorter interurinary intervals due to the organic etiology of the disorder.

A bladder training procedure can be used to deal with urinary urges. The patient can be instructed to ingest a specified amount of fluid one hour prior to each scheduled urination. The amount of fluid can be gradually increased. In a study by Figueroa and Jacob (1981), the patient started with 8 ounces of liquid and every nine days added 8 additional ounces until 32 ounces of fluid were being ingested. As a final additional aid in convincing patients that they have control over urination, and that any fear of enuresis is unfounded, patients can be instructed to remain close to home but to urinate only three to four times during the day.

Espie (1985) successfully combined the bladder training procedure with in vivo systematic desensitization to treat two cases of urinary urgency. Cognitive restructuring may be helpful in modifying any misconceptions about the problem and any fears of catastrophe.

For More Information

Figueroa, J., & Jacob, R. (1981). Treatment of urinary urgency and excessive frequency: A case study. *Behavior Research and Therapy, 19*, 261-264.

This article describes the use of urinary scheduling, relaxation training, and a bladder training procedure to treat both the urge to urinate and the frequency of urination in a single case study. The article can be obtained from Rolf Jacob, University of Pittsburgh School of Medicine, Western Psychiatric Institute and Clinic, 3811 O'Hara Street, Pittsburgh, PA 15261.

Masur, F. (1976). Behavior therapy in a case of pollakiuria. *Journal of Behavior Therapy and Experimental Psychiatry, 7*, 175-178.

This article describes the successful use of urinary scheduling in a single case study. A contingent reward and "fine" system is explained. The article can be obtained from Frank T. Masur, Highland Hospital, Division of Duke University Medical Center, Department of Psychology, Box 1101, Asheville, NC 28802.

References

Cohen, S., & Reed, J. (1968). The treatment of "nervous diarrhea" and other conditioned autonomic disorders by desensitization. *British Journal of Psychiatry, 114*, 1275-1280.

Espie, C. (1985). Treatment of excessive urinary urgency and frequency by retention control training and desensitization: Three case studies. *Behavior Research and Therapy, 23*, 205-210.

Figueroa, J., & Jacob, R. (1981). Treatment of urinary urgency and excessive frequency: A case study. *Behavior Research and Therapy, 19*, 261-264.

Masur, F. (1976). Behavior therapy in a case of pollakiuria. *Journal of Behavior Therapy and Experimental Psychiatry, 7*, 175-178.

O'Neill, G. (1982). Behavior therapy for urinary frequency in a patient with neurogenic bladder: A case report. *General Hospital Psychiatry, 4*, 15-18.

Rovetto, F. (1983). Treatment of excessive urinary frequency and urgency by desensitization and progressive retention training. *Journal of Behavior Therapy and Experimental Psychiatry, 14*, 155-159.

Yates, A., & Poole, A. (1972). Behavioral analysis in the case of excessive frequency of micturiton. *Behavior Therapy, 3*, 449-453.

42 Urinary Retention

Assessment Strategies

Initially a consultation with a physician may be necessary to rule out any organic basis for the problem. The behavioral assessment involves both in vivo and self-report measures. The patient should keep a behavioral diary composed of various measures surrounding the attempt to urinate. The diary should contain a description of the general setting and bathroom, the number of people present, an urge to urinate rating (1-10), and a SUDS rating prior to any attempt to urinate. The use of the measure of latency to urinate has been found to exacerbate the problem for some patients and therefore should be avoided as an assessment measure. In vivo assessment of at least one week is recommended.

Other self-report measures, such as the Fear Survey Schedule or the Social Avoidance and Distress Scale, may be necessary to determine if social anxiety or other phobias are present.

Treatment Strategies

A patient who scores high on social anxiety may need assertiveness training prior to, or concurrent with, any of the methods presented in this chapter.

Imaginal systematic desensitization has generally not been found to be effective in treating urinary retention (Glasgow, 1975). However, in vivo desensitization (i.e., exposure), with or without the therapist present, has been used effectively in treating this problem (e.g., Lamontagne & Marks, 1973). In applying in vivo desensitization patients are told not to urinate until the need to urinate is very high. This need can be enhanced through the consumption of beverages. Tea, a natural diuretic, is strongly recommended. When the patient is attempting an in vivo item, it is important that he or she remains in the situation until urination occurs. Practicing controlling the sphincter, by starting and stopping the flow of urine, may also be helpful. Each in vivo trial should be repeated until the patient is successful in urinating in less than ten seconds. In vivo treatment can be completed in eight to ten sessions.

Homework assignments between sessions should focus on generalization of the types and locations of bathrooms. Additionally, the behavioral diary should be continued during the treatment stage.

A combination of in vivo and imaginal exposure may be necessary for some patients (e.g., Wilson, 1973). The patient can attempt urination in a place that assures success (e.g., home). At the time when urination is inevitable, the patient can imagine someone entering the room. The imaginal scenes can be developed in the therapy sessions and practiced between sessions.

If in vivo desensitization is not successful, there is some evidence that a paradoxical technique may be helpful (Ascher, 1979). Ascher (1979) told his patients to "engage in all of the activities which were typically associated with urinating" (p. 269)—but they were prohibited from urinating.

Ascher (1979) describes the procedure as follows:

> **A male client was to enter the men's room, walk to the urinal, unzip his fly, perform the appropriate manipulation and stand there as if to urinate. Under no circumstances is he to allow himself to pass urine. After a reasonable period of time he was to readjust his anatomy, return his pants to the proper order, flush the urinal, wash his hands, and leave the bathroom. . . . Once clients reported a violation of this prohibition they were expected to attempt to inhibit the flow of urine for as long as possible each time they entered a restroom associated with anxiety. [p. 269]**

The technique appears to work rapidly, within six weeks.

For More Information

Anderson, L. (1977). Desensitization in vivo for men unable to urinate in a public facility. *Journal of Behavior Therapy and Experimental Psychiatry, 8*, 105-106.

This study describes the use of the in vivo desensitization technique with a series of five patients. The article can be obtained from Lowell Anderson, Ph.D., Department of Psychiatry, New York University Medical School, 550 First Ave., New York, NY 10016.

Ascher, L. (1979). Paradoxical intention in the treatment of urinary retention. *Behavior Research and Therapy, 17*, 267-273.

This article describes the use of paradoxical intention in a series of five cases that were unsuccessfully treated with desensitization. The article can be obtained from L. Michael Ascher, Department of Psychiatry, Temple University, Henry Ave., Philadelphia, PA 19129.

References

Ascher, L. (1979). Parodoxical intention in the treatment of urinary retention. *Behavior Research and Therapy, 17*, 267-273.

Glasgow, R. (1975). In vivo prolonged exposure in the treatment of urinary retention. *Behavior Therapy, 6*, 701-702.

Lamontagne, Y., & Marks, I. (1973). Psychogenic urinary retention: Treatment by prolonged exposure. *Behavior Therapy, 4*, 581-585.

Wilson, G. (1973). Innovations in the modification of phobic behaviors in two clinical cases. *Behavior Therapy, 4*, 426-430.

43 Vaginismus

Assessment Strategies

Vaginismus is characterized by difficulty in penile entry into the vagina due to "an involuntary contracting of the muscle around the outer third of the vagina" (Fuchs, 1980). These muscles may even contract at the thought of penile entry. A pelvic examination should precede any behavioral assessment, since there are some physical conditions that can obstruct vaginal entry.

A behavioral assessment involves taking a history of when the pain occurs and a description of the most recent attempts at intercourse. It is important to assess the patient's thoughts regarding the problem (e.g., "We will never be able to have a normal sex life"). It is also important to differentiate vaginismus from phobic avoidance of intercourse. Other areas of sexual dysfunction should also be assessed (e.g., female orgasmic dysfunction, male erection or ejaculation problems, and sexual desire).

Treatment Strategies

Education, of both the man and the woman, generally precedes any behavioral treatment. The involuntary nature of vaginismus should be explained to the patient. The use of anatomical illustrations or models may be helpful. It is useful to dispel any misconceptions about the dangerousness of penetration.

The most successful behavioral treatments are in vitro and in vivo desensitization. In vitro desensitization generally precedes in vivo if the patient has any phobic avoidance of vaginal entry. Shahar and Jaffe (1978) describe a typical hierarchy that can be used for in vitro and in vivo desensitization:

> **1. Intromission of one finger.**
> **2. Intromission of a small-size dilator.**
> **3. Intromission of two fingers.**
> **4. Intromission of a larger-size dilator.**
> **5. Partial intromission by the penis.**
> **6. Full intromission by the penis.**
> **[p. 58]**

Other items that could be added to a hierarchy include: sexual foreplay, insertion of the husband's finger, or insertion of a tampon. Hierarchy steps can also precede from the woman inserting a dilator, to inserting a dilator in the presence of the man, to the man inserting the dilator under the woman's manual control. During the in vivo exercises, Cooper (1969) recommends that if a spasm occurs "during penile penetration he should not withdraw, but should remain where he was until the spasm and associated pain disappeared, when he was to continue penetration in a leisurely and unhurried manner" (p. 722). During the initial attempts at penile insertion, Fuchs (1980) suggests that the couple be in the female superior position and that "the man is asked to be passive and allow the woman to assume the active role" (p. 4). Masters and Johnson (1970) precede the desensitization with sensate focus exercises and an initial ban on intercourse.

If the assessment reveals distorted thinking, rational restructuring can easily be added to a desensitization program.

Wilson (1973) has successfully used orgasmic re-conditioning in a single case study. Initially the patient is to:

> **Imagine minimal finger insertion immediately preceding orgasm. She was able to do this without any impairment of orgasm and was then carefully instructed to imagine gradually increasing amounts of finger insertion progressively earlier in the chain of fantasy and behavior which culminated in orgasm. Three weeks later the client was able to imagine insertion without any impairment of the development and maintenance of sexual arousal. . . . after this therapeutic advance the client was instructed to have her boyfriend begin inserting his finger into her vagina immediately prior to her achieving orgasm. In other words, the procedure she had successfully completed in fantasy was repeated at the behavioral level. [p. 428]**

Kegel exercises have also been used to teach voluntary control over the pubococcygeus muscles which are involved in vaginismus. The exercises involve: "working up to a specific maintenance level of contractions both in terms of the strength of the contraction and the rapidity with which she could squeeze the muscles in sequence" (Birk & Brinkley-Birk, 1975). The exercises are practiced daily by the patient.

For More Information

Fertel, N. (1977). Vaginismus: a review. *Journal of Sex and Marital Therapy, 3*, 113-121.

This article reviews the diagnosis, etiology, and behavioral treatment approaches to vaginismus. There is a good description of the Masters and Johnson program and the desensitization treatment. The article can be obtained from Norman Fertel, M.D., Department of Obstetrics and Gynecology, Beth Israel Hospital, 330 Brookline Avenue, Boston, MA. 02215.

Fuchs, K. (1980). Therapy of vaginismus by hypnotic desensitization. *American Journal of Obstetrics and Gynecology, 137*, 1-7.

This article describes the desensitization treatment of vaginismus. Case illustrations, including sample hierarchies, are reviewed. The article can be obtained from Dr. Carl Fuchs, Department of Obstetrics and Gynecology, Rambam Medical Center, Faculty of Medicine, Technion-Israel Institute of Technology, Haifa, Israel.

References

Birk, L., & Brinkley-Birk, A. (1975). Sex therapy of vaginismus, primary impotence and ejaculatory incompetence in an unconsummated marriage. *Psychiatric Opinion, 12*, 30.

Cooper, A. (1969). An innovation in the "behavioral" treatment of the case of non-consummation due to vaginismus. *British Journal of Psychiatry, 115*, 721-722.

Fuchs, K. (1980). Therapy of vaginismus by hypnotic desensitization. *American Journal of Obstetrics and Gyncology, 137*, 1-7.

Masters, W., & Johnson, V. (1970). *Human sexual inadequacy*. Boston: Little Brown.

Shahar, A., & Jaffe, Y. (1978). Behavior and cognitive therapy in the treatment of vaginismus: A case study. *Cognitive Therapy and Research, 2*, 57-60.

Wilson, G. (1973). Innovations in the modification of phobic behaviors in two clinical cases. *Behavior Therapy, 4*, 426-430.

44 Vomiting

Assessment Strategies

Vomiting can be a symptom of many disorders (e.g., bulimia or the side effects from cancer chemotherapy) or it can occur as the primary symptom for treatment. It is important to precede any behavioral assessment with a physical exam emphasizing gastrointestinal studies to rule out an organic cause of the vomiting. Behavioral assessment for vomiting generally involves having the patient record the frequency of the vomiting and complete a behavioral diary including antecedents and consequences of each vomiting episode. For patients who vomit after eating, an actual food trial can be set up. The patient can be observed after eating small amounts of food recommended by a dietician. Frequency of vomiting and the latency from eating to vomiting should be recorded.

Treatment Strategies

The behavioral assessment should help to pinpoint the behaviors maintaining the vomiting. If the assessment indicates the vomiting is precipitated by anxiety provoking situations, then relaxation training or systematic desensitization can be applied. Rebman (1983) utilized cue-controlled relaxation in a self-controlled desensitization procedure to eliminate vomiting associated with anxiety about air travel. In the self-controlled desensitization procedure, the patient can be instructed to write out a detailed description of the anxiety situation using a temporal hierarchy. One scene per day can be practiced for about 15 minutes. If the patient experiences anxiety during the writing, the cue-controlled relaxation can be applied.

Stravynski (1983) used social skills training as one important treatment component for a patient whose vomiting was associated with social anxiety. Burgess (1969) and Peck (1978) utilized in vivo exposure and stimulus control techniques to eliminate vomiting associated with a conditioned anxiety response. In applying the stimulus control techniques, it is necessary to change the stimuli pattern and cues that normally lead to the vomiting response. For example, after discovering that vomiting occurred only at bedtime, Peck (1978) altered her patient's bedtime routine by changing the time she went to bed, the bathroom used, and the general order of her bedtime routine.

Latimer, Malmed, and Fisher (1982) have used exposure and response prevention successfully to treat vomiting. In applying these techniques, the patient is asked to eat and then encouraged not to vomit. Each treatment session involves larger and more difficult foods based on the patient's ratings. Toward the end of treatment the patient can be instructed to do things that could make him or her more likely to vomit (e.g., walking immediately after eating). During the treatment it is important that the patient not be provided with any facilities for emesis.

Welch (1979) found a response delay strategy in combination with response prevention and cognitive restructuring sucessful in eliminating self-induced vomiting in one patient. Welch (1979) describes the procedure as follows:

> **Time graduated response delay was accomplished by asking Mrs. B how long she believed she could wait at the following steps in the forced vomiting response chain: (1) after finding, but before entering a restroom; (2) after entering the restroom; (3) after kneeling or bending over the toilet bowl; and (4) after the finger was inserted. One minute at each step was the agreed upon starting time period. With each successful week the time period was increased. The amount of increase was at each point determined by Mrs. B. [p. 79]**

Thought stopping can be used to deal with any obsessive thoughts that occur preceding or subsequent to the vomiting. Additionally, cognitive restructuring may be helpful for some patients.

An alternative counter-conditioning strategy involves pairing ginger ale with the stimuli that elicit the vomiting. Ginger ale in small amounts (5 cc) provides normal peristaltic activity of the stomach and small intestines which is incompatible with vomiting. To insure that all the stimuli associated with vomiting are covered, the patient can be asked to take sips of ginger ale every 15 minutes during the entire day. It may also be important to utilize other behaviors that have been found to be incompatible with the patient's vomiting. For example, Stoffelmayer (1970) found that reading out loud at a rapid pace was incompatible with his patient's retching and gagging responses. Emotive (pleasant) imagery can also be used at the time any nausea is felt (Tasto & Chesney, 1977). The technique can first be applied in imagination by having the patient imagine stimuli that cause nausea and then transferring to in vivo situations. If the assessment indicates that the vomiting is maintained by attention and social contact, then an extinction procedure should be attempted. Any conversation about vomiting or nausea should be ignored and a time-out procedure should be applied to any actual vomiting episode. It is necessary to reinforce more adaptive, incompatible behavior if extinction techniques are used.

With the adult mentally retarded patient, a positive practice and self-correction procedure is recommended (Azrin & Wesolowski, 1975). Self-correction requires that the patient clean up the vomiting and change any clothes or bedsheets that have been soiled. Following self-correction, the patient can engage in 15 positive practice trials. The positive practice requires that the patient be taken to the toilet, bend over with his or her mouth open for several seconds, and then flush the toilet. The patient is then taken back to the scene where the vomiting occurred, and the next positive practice trial is initiated. It may also be important to remind the patient throughout the day of where to vomit and the consequences of not vomiting in the correct place. It may take a week before any results are seen using this technique.

Duker and Seys (1977) added positive reinforcement (e.g., attention or bodily contact) for non-vomiting behavior to an over-correction procedure in successfully reducing vomiting in a profoundly retarded adult.

Food satiation has also been used successfully to reduce vomiting in two profoundly retarded adults. Jackson, Johnson, Ackron, and Crowley (1975) describe the procedure as follows:

> **The food-satiation treatment condition consisted of allowing the subject to eat all of the food he could consume. Food satiation was achieved by allowing the subject to eat double portions of the standard meal, in addition to cereal, ice cream, and milk shakes. The criterion for satiation was the refusal of food twice with a 1-minute interval between the food refusals. In the event that the subject left the dining room table, he was returned to the table and again offered the food. If the subject exhibited an eating response upon returning to the meal, the satiation criterion was again in effect. Immediately after each 1-hour recording session, throughout the treatment conditions, the subject was offered .53 l of milkshake to maintain the effect of satiation throughout the day. A maintenance procedure was initiated immediately after the second treatment condition in which the subject received double portions of the standard meal at scheduled meal times. [p. 224]**

Relaxation combined with stimulus deprivation has been successfully used in treating vomiting in a pregnant patient (Simone & Cong, 1985). Stimulus deprivation consisted of placing the patient in a relatively stimulus-free environment for a period of three days.

The use of aversive conditioning with shock has been shown to be successful in one case study of an adult mentally retarded patient who evidenced vomiting (Kohlenberg, 1979).

Psychogenic regurgitation may require different treatment than vomiting. Esophagol training, as used in speech therapy, has been shown to be helpful for this problem. The training involves ingesting carbonated beverages, doing sit-up exercises, and "externally applying abdominal pressure in order to distend the esophagus and force the patient to control the passage of contents from the stomach to the esophagus" (Krajewski, 1980; p. 265).

For More Information

Mogan, J., & O'Brien, J. (1972). The counter conditioning of a vomiting habit by sips of ginger ale. *Journal of Behavior Therapy and Experimental Psychiatry, 3*, 135-137.

This article describes the use of ginger ale as a counter conditioning agent for vomiting in a single case study. The article can be obtained from John S. O'Brien, 17 Henshaw Street, Brighton, MA 02135.

Peck, C. (1978). Modification of a learned vomiting ritual by change in stimulus condition and self-controlled response prevention. *Journal of Behavior Therapy and Experimental Psychiatry, 9*, 359-363.

his article describes the use of a response prevention procedure, stimulus control techniques, and in vivo desensitization in the successful treatment of a single case of conditioned vomiting. The article can be obtained from Connie L. Peck, Department of Psychology, La Trobe University, Bundoora, Victoria, 3083, Australia.

References

Azrin, N., & Wesolowski, M. (1975). Eliminating habitual vomiting in a retarded adult by positive practice and self-correction. *Journal of Behavior Ther-*

apy and Experimental Psychiatry, 6, 145-148.

Burgess, E. (1969). Elimination of vomiting behavior. *Behavior Research and Therapy, 11*, 173-176.

Duker, P., & Seys, D. (1977). Elimination of vomiting in a retarded female using restitutional overcorrection. *Behavior Therapy, 8*, 255-257.

Jackson, G., Johnson, C., Ackron, G., & Crowley, R. (1975). Food satiation as a procedure to decelerate vomiting. *American Journal of Mental Deficiency, 80*, 223-227.

Kohlenberg, R. (1970). The punishment of persistent vomiting: A case study. *Journal of Applied Behavioral Analysis, 3*, 241-245.

Krajewski, J. (1980). Psychogenic regurgitation: A specific entity and suggested treatment. *Journal of Behavior Therapy and Experimental Psychiatry, 11*, 263-266.

Latimer, P., Malmud, L., & Fisher, R. (1982). Gastric stasis and vomiting: Behavioral treatment. *Gastroenterology, 83*, 684-688.

Peck, C. (1978). Modification of a learned vomiting ritual by changing stimulus conditions and self-controlled response prevention. *Journal of Behavior Therapy and Experimental Psychiatry, 9*, 359-363.

Rebman, V. (1983). Self-control desensitization with cue controlled relaxation for treatment of a conditioned vomiting response to air travel. *Journal of Behavior Therapy and Experimental Psychiatry, 14*, 161-164.

Simone, S., & Long, M. (1985). The behavioral treatment of hyperemesis gravidarum. *The Behavior Therapist, 8*, 128-129.

Stoffelmayer, B. (1970). The treatment of a retching response to dentures by counteractive reading aloud. *Journal of Behavior Therapy and Experimental Psychiatry, 1*, 163-164.

Stravynski, A. (1983). Behavioral treatment of psychogenic vomiting in the context of social phobia. *Journal of Nervous and Mental Disease, 171*, 448-451.

Tasto, D., & Chesney, M. (1977). The deconditioning of nausea and of crying by emotive imagery: A report of two case studies. *Journal of Behavior Therapy and Experimental Psychiatry, 8*, 139-142.

Welch, G. (1979). The treatment of compulsive vomiting and obsessive thoughts through graduated response delay, response prevention, and cognitive correction. *Journal of Behavior Therapy and Experimental Psychiatry, 10*, 77-82.

See Also

Chapter 6. Bulimia
Chapter 8. Cancer

45 Writer's Cramp

Assessment Strategies

Writer's cramp is a movement disorder characterized by muscle spasm, a lack of coordination, and often pain when an individual attempts to write. Any behavioral assessment should be preceded by a medical or neurological evaluation, or both.

A pretreatment assessment can consist of some very simple measures. The patient should rate both the severity of interference with normal activities and the amount of discomfort experienced on a "0-to-8" scale, with 8 indicating the greatest severity. Initial measurements that can also be used during treatment include: a simple count of the number of cramps per minute, the latency between the cramps, or the number of words written per minute. It may also be helpful to take these measures in an environment in which the problem is more likely to be evident.

For some patients, writer's cramp has been associated with a high degree of anxiety, unexpressed anger, or both. Therefore, a general measure of anxiety (e.g., State-Trait Anxiety Inventory) and assertiveness (e.g., Rathus Assertiveness Schedule) can be included in the basic assessment.

Treatment Strategies

A combination of graduated exposure, habit reversal, and re-education may work very rapidly in the majority of patients. Greenberg (1983) describes some modifications of the habit reversal technique when used with patients with writer's cramp. During the "awareness training" the patient and the therapist develop a list of situations in which writer's cramp may occur. Then, the cramp is defined by both the patient and the therapist and demonstrated by the therapist to the patient. Next, while observing the patient, the therapist tells the patient when a cramp has started. During "habit-reversal practice," the therapist demonstrates an incompatible response and then the patient attempts the response. As an example of an incompatible response, Greenberg (1983) uses an extension of the thumb, fingers, and wrist of the writing hand when a spasm occurs or is about to start. This movement is maintained for 5 to 10 seconds. A significant other in the patient's home environment should be used to provide social reinforcement to encourage and supervise practice and discourage any attempts to write with the opposite hand.

Re-education procedures are often preceded by relaxation training. The relaxation training focuses on the arm, hand, and fingers of the writing hand. It may be especially important to relax the grip of the writing instrument and equalize the pressure of the fingers that are responsible for holding the writing instrument. Re-education involves the use of different writing instruments and different tasks. The progression of writing instruments may begin with a watercolor-sized paintbrush and proceed to a broad felt-tipped pen, a soft pencil, a hard pencil, a sketch pen, and finally an ordinary pen. With each writing instrument, the patient should master a series of tasks beginning with simply making contact with the paper. The writing tasks then progress to drawing large circles, then smaller circles, then spirals, then horizontal and vertical lines. Finally letters and words are practiced. At each practice session the size of the writing is reduced. For some patients the initial session may have to be conducted with a supinated hand. Once all the tasks are mastered with the supinated hand, the patient should attempt writing with the hand in a normal writing position. During practice, patients should be instructed to stop the task if they feel any pain. After mastering the task during the session, a half hour of home practice should be assigned. There should be no other writing outside the session or practice unless absolutely necessary. This type of retraining program may take anywhere from one to four months.

Systematic desensitization, or in vivo exposure, may be necessary to deal with the anxiety that has been associated with writing. In using these techniques the patient attempts writing in a hierarchical series of tasks. The items on the hierarchy consist of situations in which the cramp is likely to occur. Each situation on the hierarchy should be assigned a SUDS rating by the patient and then the tasks should be assigned in ascending order. Patients using this technique should be instructed to stop writing whenever pain or discomfort is felt and immediately to use relaxation training for a few minutes.

Combined habit reversal, retraining, and in vivo exposure may substantially cut down the overall length of treatment. With the combined treatment results may be seen in three to seven hours of therapy.

Sanavio (1982) successfully used a combination of extinction and response prevention in treating two patients with writer's cramp. He describes the procedure as follows:

> **Subjects were instructed to perform the task without resorting to escape behaviors and to maintain paper and pen contact until the signal for the rest period. Escape behaviors were punished by extending the duration of the (aversive) task period to a maximum of 50 sec and curtailing the rest period. During this treatment phase the subjects were encouraged to deal with tension fluctuations and cramps in a relaxed manner rather than their accustommed escape behaviors. . . . The degree of difficulty of the task was gradually increased. Treatment variations included extending the period of pen and paper contact from 25 sec to 5 min, using different pens in increasingly difficult writing exercises and assigned homework. [p. 71]**

For some patients the use of assertion training or anger control techniques may be needed if the assessment shows that these problems are related to the occurrence of the writer's cramp.

Uchiyana, Lutteijohann, and Shah (1977) successfully combined biofeedback of the muscles that become tense during writing with systematic desensitization to treat successfully two patients.

Although there were some early reports of the successful use of aversive (electrical shock) conditioning techniques, the results have not been supported by more recent studies. In fact, aversive conditioning may exacerbate the problem for some patients. This is especially true when the patient has a high level of anxiety at the beginning.

For More Information

Beech, C. (1960). The symptomatic treatment of writer's cramp. In H. Eysenck (Ed.), *Behavior Therapy and the Neuroses*, pp. 349-372. New York: Pergamon Press.

This chapter presents an excellent description of the disorder and a discussion of three different treatment techniques: avoidance conditioning, negative practice, and reciprocal inhibition. Four case studies are presented that demonstrate the different clinical strategies and their effectiveness. The book can be obtained from Pergamon Press Inc., Maxwell House, Fairview Park, Elmsford, NY 10523.

Greenberg, D. (1983). Writer's cramp - a habit for reversal? *Journal of Behavior Therapy and Experimental Psychiatry, 14*, 233-239.

This article describes the use of the combined treatment approach of habit reversal, in vivo exposure, and re-education with four individual cases. The article contains a good summary of the outcome of previous studies. The article can be obtained from David Greenberg, Jerusalem Mental Health Center, Ezrat Nashin, Givat Shaul, P.O.B. 140, Jerusalem, Israel.

References

Greenberg, D. (1983). Writer's cramp - a habit for reversal? *Journal of Behavior Therapy and Experimental Psychiatry, 14*, 233-239.

Sanavio, E. (1982). An operant approach to the treatment of writer's cramp. *Journal of Behavior Therapy and Experimental Psychiatry, 13*, 69-72.

Uchiyana, K., Lutteijohann, M., & Shah, M. (1977). Biofeedback-assisted desensitization treatment of writer's cramp. *Journal of Behavior Therapy and Experimental Psychiatry, 8*, 169-171.

See Also

Chapter 30. Pain - Chronic

Appendix A: *Case Studies*

Excessive Daytime Sleepiness

Reference: Kolko, D. (1984). Behavioral treatment of excessive daytime sleepiness in an elderly woman with multiple medical problems. *Journal of Behavior Therapy and Experimental Psychiatry, 15*, 341-345.

Assessment Technique: Functional analysis of the patient's sleep attacks; including frequency, antecedents and consequences.

Treatment Technique: Progressive muscle relaxation and fluid restriction to facilitate sleep maintenance and rubber-band aversion to facilitate daytime arousal.

Hives

Reference: Daniels, L. (1973). Treatment of urticaria and severe headache by behavior therapy. *Psychosomatics, 14*, 347-351.

Assessment Technique: Patient observation of hives.

Treatment Technique: Systematic desensitization to deal with anxiety arousing situations, thought-stopping to inhibit acute anxiety, and covert reinforcement to increase good feelings following the thought stopping.

Muscle Spasm

Reference: Butler, P., & Salamy, A. (1975). Eliminating a conditioned muscle spasm by an electric vibrator. *Journal of Behavior Therapy and Experimental Psychiatry, 6*, 159-161.

Assessment Technique: Behavior diary to determine under what conditions the muscle spasm occurs.

Treatment Technique: Systematic desensitization, with the application of a hand-held vibrator to the specific muscle group. Vibrator is eventually faded out of the treatment.

Polydipsia

Reference: Klonoff, E., & Moore, D. (1984). Compulsive polydipsia presenting as diabetes insipidus: A behavioral approach. *Journal of Behavior Therapy and Experimental Psychiatry, 15*, 353-358.

Assessment Technique: Medical evaluation. Nursing observation of fluids ingested and time and amount of urinary output. Self-monitoring of drinking, urinating, and urges.

Treatment Technique: Response prevention, frontalis EMG biofeedback and removal of social reinforcement for drinking.

Psoriasis

Reference: Waxman, D. (1973). Behavior therapy of psoriasis: A hypnoanalytic and counter-conditioning technique. *Post-Graduate Medical Journal, 49*, 591-595.

Assessment Technique: Observation of patient's affected areas.

Treatment Technique: Relaxation-hypnosis, imagined and in vivo systematic desensitization, and assertion training.

Sleeptalking

Reference: Le Boeuf, A. (1979). A behavioral treatment of chronic sleeptalking. *Journal of Behavior Therapy and Experimental Psychiatry, 10*, 83-84.

Assessment Technique: Tape recorder with microphone on bedroom table.

Treatment Technique: Aversive tone presented for 5 seconds contingent on vocalization.

Sleep-walking

Reference: Meyer, R. (1975). A behavioral treatment of sleepwalking associated with test anxiety. *Journal of Behavior Therapy and Experimental Psychiatry, 6*, 167-168.

Assessment Technique: Monitored by wife.

Treatment Technique: Loud whistle contingent on sleepwalking.

Speaking Stomach Syndrome

Reference: Bleisenberg, G., & Cluysenaer, S. (1983). Behavioral treatment of the speaking stomach syndrome. *Journal of Behavior Medicine, 6*, 115-122.

Assessment Technique: Patient record of amount of time problem occurs per day and patient rating of the intensity of the complaint.

Treatment Technique: Breathing retraining.

Vertigo

Reference: Fowler, R., Chawla, N., Lehmann, J., & Tindall, V. (1971). An application of behavior therapy to a program of debilitating vertigo. *Behavior Therapy, 2*, 589-591.

Assessment Technique: Degree of elevation from bed, graphed and displayed.

Treatment Technique: Extinction for sick behaviors and reinforcement for well behaviors.

Permissions

Chapter 1

Table 1-1 from Garner, D., & Garfinkel, P. (1979). The Eating Attitudes Test: An index of the symptoms of anorexia nervosa. *Psychological Medicine, 9*, 278. Copyrighted and reprinted with permission of Cambridge University Press.

Table 1-2 from Slade, P. (1973). A short anorexic behavior scale. *British Journal of Psychiatry, 122*, 83. Reprinted with permission of the publisher.

Passage from Mavissakalian, M. (1982). Anorexia nervosa treated with response prevention and prolonged exposure. *Behavior Research and Therapy, 20*, 28. Reprinted with permission of Pergamon Press, Inc. and the author.

Chapter 2

Table 2-1 from Nimmer, W., & Kapp, R. (1974). A multiple impact program for the treatment of injection phobias. *Journal of Behavior Therapy and Experimental Psychiatry, 5*, 258. Reprinted with permission of Pergamon Press, Inc. and the author.

Passage from Taylor, C.B., Ferguson, M., & Wermuth, B.M. (1977). Simple techniques to treat medical phobias. In *Postgraduate Medical Journal, 53*, 28-32. Reprinted with permission of Macmillan & Company and the author.

Passage from Elmore, R., Wildman, R., & Westfield, J. (1980). The use of systematic desensitization in the treatment of blood phobia. *Journal of Behavior Therapy and Experimental Psychiatry, 11*, 278. Reprinted with permission of Pergamon Press, Inc. and the author.

Chapter 4

Tables 4-1 and 4-2 from Erskine, J., & Schonell, M. (1979). Relaxation therapy in bronchial asthma. *Journal of Psychosomatic Research, 23*, 131-139. Adapted with permission of Pergamon Press, Inc.

Passage from Sirota, A., & Mahoney, M. (1974). Relaxing on cue: The self regulation of asthma. *Journal of Behavior Therapy and Experimental Psychiatry, 5*, 65-66. Reprinted with permission of Pergamon Press, Inc. and the author.

Passage from Yorkston, N., McHugh, R., Serber, M., & Sergeant, H. (1974). Verbal desensitization in bronchial asthma. *Journal of Psychosomatic Research, 18*, 372-373. Reprinted with permission of Pergamon Press, Inc.

Chapter 6

Passages from Leitenberg, H., Gross, J., Peterson, J., & Rosen, J. (1984). Analysis of an anxiety model in the process of change during exposure plus response prevention in the treatment of bulimia nervosa. *Behavior Therapy, 15*, 6-9. Copyright 1984 by the Association for the Advancement of Behavior Therapy. Reprinted by permission of the publisher and the authors.

Table 6-1 from Hawkins, R., & Clement, P. (1980). Development and construct validation of a self-report measure of binge eating tendencies. *Addictive Behaviors, 5*, 219-226. Reprinted with permission of Pergamon Press, Inc. and the author.

Passage from Schneider, J., & Agras, W. (1985). A cognitive behavioural group treatment of bulimia. *British Journal of Psychiatry, 146*, 67-68. Reprinted with permission of the publisher and the authors.

Chapter 10

Passage from Shelton, J., & Levy, R. (1981). *Behavioral assignments and treatment compliance: A handbook of clinical strategies*, p. 49. Reprinted with permission of Research Press.

Chapter 12

Passage from Malmo, R.B., Davis, J.F., & Barza, S. (1952). Total hysterical deafness: An experimental case study. *Journal of Personality, 21*(2), 195. Copyright 1953 Duke University Press. Reprinted with permission of the publisher.

Chapter 13

Figure 13-1, Dental Anxiety Scale. From Corah, N. (1969). Devleopment of a dental anxiety scale. *Journal of Dental Research, 48*, 596. Reprinted with permission of the American Association of Dental Research.

Figure 13-2, Dental Fear Survey. From Kleinknecht, R., Klepac, R., & Alexander, J. (1973). Origins and characteristics of fear of dentistry. *Journal of the American Dental Association., 86*, 844-845. Copyright by the American Dental Association. Reprinted by permission.

Figure 13-3, Hierarchy for Systematic Desensitization. From Gale, E., & Ayer, W. (1969). Treatment of dental phobias. *Journal of the American Dental Association, 78*, 1306. Copyright by the American Dental Association. Reprinted by permission.

Passages from Jerremalm, A., Janson, L., & Ost, L. (1986). Individual response patterns and the effects of different behavioral methods in the treatment of dental phobia. *Behavior Research and Therapy, 24*, 590-591. Reprinted with permission of Pergamon Press and the authors.

Passages from Kleinknecht, R., & Bernstein, D. (1979). Short term therapy of dental avoidance. *Journal of Behavior Therapy and Experimental Psychiatry, 10*, 311-312. Reprinted with permission of Pergamon Press and the authors.

Chapter 14

Table 14-1 from Fowler, J., Budzynski, T., & VandenBergh, R. (1976). Effects of an EMG biofeedback relaxation program on the control of diabetes. *Biofeedback and Self-Regulation, 1*, 108. Reprinted with permission of Plenum Publishing Company.

Chapter 16

Passage from Denney, D., & Gerrard, M. (1981). Behavioral treatments of primary dysmenorrhea: A review. *Behavior Research and Therapy, 19*, 309. Reprinted with permission of Pergamon Press and the authors.

Passage from Cox, D., & Meyer, R. (1978). Behavioral treatment parameters with primary dysmenorrhea. *Journal of Behavioral Medicine, 1*, 301. Reprinted with permission of Plenum Publishing Corporation and the authors.

Passage from Chesney, M., & Tasto, D. (1975). The effectiveness of behavior modification with spasmodic and congestive dysmenorrhea. *Behavior Research and Therapy, 13*, 248. Reprinted from Pergamon Press and the authors.

Passage from Quillen, M., & Denney, D. (1982). Self-control of dysmenorrheic symptoms through pain management training. *Journal of Behavior Therapy and Experimental Psychiatry, 13*, 125. Reprinted with permission of Pergamon Press and the authors.

Chapter 17

Passages from Ost, L., Lindhal, I., Sterner, U., & Gerremalm, A. (1984). Exposure in vivo versus applied relaxation in the treatment of blood phobia. *Behavior Research and Therapy, 22*, 207-209. Reprinted with permission of Pergamon Press and the authors.

Passage from McGrady, A., & Bernal, G. (1986). Relaxation based treatment of a stress-induced syncopy. *Journal of Behavior Therapy and Experimental Psychiatry, 17*, 26. Reprinted with permission of Pergamon Press and the author.

Passage from Wardle, J., & Jarvis, M. (1981). The paradoxical fear response to blood, injury and illness—a treatment report. *Behavioural Psychotherapy, 9*, 16.

Reprinted with permission of the British Association of Behavioural Psychotherapy.

Chapter 19

Passage from Blanchard, E., & Andrasik, F. (1984). *Management of chronic headaches, a psychological approach*, pp. 15-18. Reprinted with permission of Pergamon Press and the authors.

Table 19-1, Headache Frequency Record. From Bakal, D., & Kaganov, J. (1976). A simple method for self-observation of headache frequency, intensity and location. *Headache, 16*, 124. Reprinted with permission of the American Association for the Study of Headache and the authors.

Chapter 22

Passage from Bonn, J., Readhead, C., & Timmons, B. (1984). Enhanced adaptive behavioral response in agoraphobic patients pre-treated with breathing retraining. *The Lancet, 8404*, p. 666. Reprinted with permission of Lancet Ltd. and the authors.

Chapter 23

Passage from Wagner, B., & Paul, G. (1970). Reduction of incontinence in chronic mental patients: A pilot project. *Journal of Behavior Therapy and Experimental Psychiatry, 1*, 31. Reprinted with permission of Pergamon Press and the authors.

Table 23-1, Dry-Bed Procedure, from Azrin, N., Sneed, T., & Foxx, R. (1971). A rapid method of eliminating bed wetting (enuresis) of the retarded. *Behavior Research and Therapy, 11*, 430. Reprinted with permission of Pergamon Press and the authors.

Passage from Phibbs, J., & Wells, M. (1982). The treatment of nocturnal enuresis in institutionalized retarded adults. *Journal of Behavior Therapy and Experimental Psychiatry, 13*, 247. Reprinted with permission of Pergamon Press and the author.

Table 23-2, Outline of the Toilet Training Procedure, from Azrin, N., & Foxx, R. (1971). A rapid method of toilet training the institutionalized retarded. *Journal of Applied Behavior Analysis, 4*, 91. Copyright 1971 by the Society for the Experimental Analysis of Behavior, Inc. Reprinted with permission of the publisher and authors.

Chapter 24

Passage from Bootzin, R. (1977). *Behavioral treatment of insomnia: A clinician's guide and self-management techniques for controlling insomnia*. Reprinted with permission of BMA Audiocasette Programs.

Passage from Stam, H., & Butz, B. (1986). The treatment of severe insomnia in a cancer patient. *Journal of Behavior Therapy and Experimental Psychiatry, 17*, 34-35. Reprinted with permission of Pergamon Press and the authors.

Chapter 26

Passage from Stevenson, D., & Delprato, D. (1983). Multiple component self-control program for menopausal hot flashes. *Journal of Behavior Therapy and Experimental Psychiatry, 14*, 138. Reprinted with permission of Pergamon Press and the authors.

Chapter 28

Passage from Rosenbaum, M., & Ayllon, T. (1981). The behavioral treatment of neurodermatitis through habit-reversal. *Behavior Research and Therapy, 19*, 315. Reprinted with permission of Pergamon Press and the author.

Chapter 29

Passage from Hamberger, L. (1982). Reduction of generalized aversive responding in a post-treatment cancer patient: Relaxation as an active coping skill. *Journal of Behavior Therapy and Experimental Psychiatry, 13*, 230-231. Reprinted with permission of Pergamon Press and the author.

Passages from Fordyce, W., Brockway, J., & Spengler, D. (1986). Acute back pain: A control-group comparison of behavioral vs traditional management methods. *Journal of Behavioral Medicine, 9*, 130-132. Reprinted with permission of Plenum Publishing Corporation and the authors.

Chapter 30

Passsage from Blinchik, E., & Grzesiak, R. (1979). Reinterpretive cognitive strategies in chronic pain management. *Archives of Physical Medical Rehabilitation, 60*, 610-611. Reprinted with permission of the American Congress of Physical Medical Rehabilitation.

Passage from Grzesiak, R. (1977). Relaxation techniques in the treatment of chronic pain. *Archives of Physical Medical Rehabilitation, 58*, 270. Reprinted with permission of the American Congress of Physical Medical Rehabilitation.

Passage from Khatami, M., & Rush, A. (1978). A pilot study of the treatment of outpatients with chronic pain: Symptom control, stimulus control and social system intervention. *Pain, 5*, 163-165. Reprinted with permission of Elsevier Science Publishers and the authors.

Passage from Cautela, J. (1977). The use of covert conditioning in modifying pain behavior. *Journal of Behavior Therapy and Experimental Psychiatry, 8*, 49. Reprinted with permission of Pergamon Press and the author.

Passage from Fordyce, W., Fowler, R., Lehmann, J., DeLateur, B., Sand, P., & Trieschmann, R. (1973). Operant conditioning in the treatment of chronic pain. *Archives of Physical Medical Rehabilitation, 58*, 403. Reprinted with permission of the American Congress of Physical Medical Rehabilitation.

Chapter 32

Passage from Forster, F., Paulsen, U., & Baughman, F. (1969). *Neurology, 19*, 719-720. Reprinted with permission of Modern Medicine Publications, Inc. and the authors.

Passage from Cautela, J., & Flannery, R. (1973). Seizures: Controlling the uncontrollable. *Journal of Rehabilitation, 39*, 34-35. Reprinted with permission of the National Rehabilitation Association.

Passage from Wells, K., Turner, S., Bellack, A., & Hersen, M. (1978). Effects of cue-controlled relaxation on psychomotor seizures: An experimental analysis. *Behavior Research and Therapy, 16*, 51. Reprinted with permission of Pergamon Press and the authors.

Passage from Daniels, L. (1975). Treatment of grand mal epilepsy by covert and operant conditioning techniques: A case study. *Psychosomatics, 16*, 66. Reprinted with permission of the Academy of Psychosomatic Medicine.

Chapter 33

Passage from Erickson, R., & Huber, H. (1975). Elimination of hysterical torticollis through the use of a metronome in an operant conditioning paradigm. *Behavior Therapy, 6*, 405-406. Reprinted with permission of Academic Press and the author.

Chapter 35

Passage from Stam, H., McGrath, P., & Brook, R. (1984). The treatment of temporomandibular joint syndrome through control of anxiety. *Journal of Behavior Therapy and Experimental Psychiatry, 15*, 43. Reprinted with permission of Pergamon Press and the authors.

Chapter 36

Table 36-1, Description of the Competing Reaction for Various Tics. From Azrin, N., Nunn, R., & Frantz, S. (1980). Habit reversal versus negative practice treatment of nervous tics. *Behavior Therapy, 11*, 174. Copyright 1980 by the

Association for the Advancement of Behavior Therapy. Reprinted by permission of the publisher and the author.

Chapter 37

Reprinted from Marlowe, F. (1973). Effective treatment of tinnitus through hypnotherapy. *American Journal of Clinical Hypnosis, 15*, 162-163. Reprinted with permission of the publisher.

Chapter 39

Table 39-1, Framingham Questionnaire. From Haynes, S., Feinleiv, N., Levine, S., Scotch, N., & Kannel, W. (1978). The relationship of psychosocial factors to coronary heart disease in the Framingham Study: Prevalence of coronary heart disease. *American Journal of Epidemiology, 107*, 384-402. Reprinted with permission of the publisher.

Chapter 43

Passage from Wilson, G. (1973). Innovations in the modification of phobic behaviors in two clinical cases. *Behavior Therapy, 4*, 428. Reprinted with permission of Academic Press and the author.

Chapter 44

Passage from Jackson, G., Johnson, C., Ackron, G., & Crowley, R. (1975). Food satiation as a procedure to decelerate vomiting. *American Journal of Mental Deficiency, 80*, 224. Reprinted with permission of the American Association of Mental Deficiency.

Chapter 45

Passage from Sanavio, E. (1982). An operant approach to the treatment of writer's cramp. *Journal of Behavior Therapy and Experimental Psychiatry, 14*, 71. Reprinted with permission of Pergamon Press and the author.

Author Index

Subject Index